AUTOPSY OF
A SUICIDAL MIND

BOOKS BY EDWIN S. SHNEIDMAN

Deaths of Man (1973)

Voices of Death (1980)

Definition of Suicide (1985)

The Suicidal Mind (1996)

Comprehending Suicide (2001)

EDITED BOOKS

Thematic Test Anaylsis (1951)

Clues to Suicide (1957)
WITH N. L. FARBEROW

The Cry for Help (1961)
WITH N. L. FARBEROW

Essays in Self-Destruction (1967)

On the Nature of Suicide (1969)

The Psychology of Suicide (1970, 1994)
WITH N. L. FARBEROW AND R. E. LITMAN

Death and the College Student (1972)

Suicide: Contemporary Developments (1976)

Death: Current Perspectives (1976, 1980, 1984)

*Endeavors in Psychology: Selections from
the Personology of Henry A. Murray* (1981)

Suicide Thoughts and Reflections, 1960–1980 (1981)

Suicide as Psychache (1993)

AUTOPSY OF
A SUICIDAL

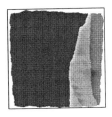

MIND

EDWIN S. SHNEIDMAN, Ph.D.

OXFORD
UNIVERSITY PRESS

2004

OXFORD
UNIVERSITY PRESS

Oxford   New York
Auckland   Bangkok   Buenos Aires   Cape Town   Chennai
Dar es Salaam   Delhi   Hong Kong   Istanbul   Karachi   Kolkata
Kuala Lumpur   Madrid   Melbourne   Mexico City   Mumbai   Nairobi
São Paulo   Shanghai   Taipei   Tokyo   Toronto

Copyright © 2004 by Edwin S. Shneidman

Published by Oxford University Press, Inc.
198 Madison Avenue, New York, New York 10016

www.oup.com

Oxford is a registered trademark of Oxford University Press

Library of Congress Cataloging-in-Publication Data
Shneidman, Edwin S.
Autopsy of a suicidal mind / Edwin S. Shneidman.
p. cm.
Includes bibliographical references.
ISBN 978-0-19-517273-7
1. Suicide—Case studies. 2. Psychological autopsy. I. Title.
RC569 .S468   2004
616.85'844509—dc22   2003016303

Printed in the United States of America
on acid-free paper

To Arthur's family—

who lent their hearts to this project

Hic locus est ubi mors gaudet succurrere vitae.

[This is the place where death rejoices in helping the living.]

—Motto above the door of the Anatomical Institute, Vienna,

where autopsies are performed.

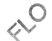

FOREWORD

I learned of Dr. Edwin Shneidman's work in suicide recovery when I was reading everything I could get my hands on about suicide after the death of my son in 1992. Dr. Shneidman's compassionate writing helped me along the way to healing, acceptance, and some degree of understanding.

Following the 10th anniversary of my son's death, and after reading many books written by Dr. Shneidman, I was writing my own book about my experience with suicide and wanted to talk to Dr. Shneidman in person. I reached out to the good doctor through friends at the university at which he has long been professor emeritus. As we talked on the phone, I came to know a little of a man who, although he has never personally lost a family member or a friend to suicide, has been intrigued, inspired, and curious about the subject of suicide for more than 60 years.

Shneidman's life work in the field of suicide, its causes, and its ramifications for survivors began when he was a young clinical psychologist. In 1949, Shneidman was asked to look at a pair of suicide notes and communicate to the widows of the men who had written them. The experience of the suicide notes, back in 1949, was so remarkable to Shneidman that he and his colleagues, Dr. Norman Farberow and Dr. Robert Litman, did the first study on suicide notes following scientific protocols. Shneidman, with his colleagues Litman and Farberow, founded the Los Angeles Suicide Prevention Center. Shneidman went on to develop a program in suicide prevention for the National Institute of Mental Health, and, eventually, to teach, write, study, and publish a number of books about suicide and contribute to many more, as well as to write seven pages of text on suicide for the 1973 edition of the *Encyclopedia Britannica*.

A few months after our first talk on the phone, I visited the doctor in Los Angeles. He sent me a note with the address and phone number and a small, exact map showing where I might find him. On the bottom of the note, he wrote, in his delicate and legible hand, "I'll leave the light on."

And, of course, that is what Professor Shneidman does. He turns on the light and leaves it shining on the hidden shadows of suicide, for all of us to see, to shed his insight so that he may help us. His light, and that of many who heal and communicate about this strange and misunderstood act of human destruction, is much needed.

Shneidman is a man whose skill and determination is matched by his compassion and articulate ability to write and communicate about the mysteries of suicide. When he began his studies as a young man, the word *suicide* was seldom more than a whisper, if ever spoken at all. Suicide and its manifestations are, by all accounts, caused by differences and problems in the brain and the emotions; chemicals such as serotonin are not found in the same levels in those who kill themselves as in those who do not. There may be spiritual, as well as physical, reasons for suicide, but most professionals and those who study the subject agree that mental illness, depression, mental pain, and even genetic patterns are probably at the root of most suicides.

At the age of 33, my son Clark died of carbon monoxide poisoning, leaving me and the rest of his family to put the pieces of our lives back together. Most of us didn't have a clue as to how we would do that. At first, I thought I, too, would die; then I realized I would have to live and didn't know how. I had to learn about the history of this traumatic taboo that haunts survivors and those who contemplate suicide. As I grieved, and read, and talked to those who knew of suicide, I learned— sometimes, it seemed, too much.

For centuries, suicide has been shrouded in secrecy. The families of suicide victims have been punished, often relieved of their possessions, sometimes rejected by their communities, the pain of their terrible loss belittled and misunderstood by friends, families, churches, and nations. It has taken courage, decades of understanding, and the steady work of compassionate professionals and everyday survivors to help professionals in therapeutic, spiritual, and community services to realize that the survivors of those who commit suicide must be treated with the same kindness and humanity as those whose loved ones may have died of diseases or been killed in sudden accidents, deaths that bring great sorrow but not the shame that has often surrounded death by self-murder. Shneidman's lifetime of work in suicide prevention and recovery has led him to the theory that, although there may be other factors, the element of "psychache" in a potential suicide may be the most important factor, one that leads to the questions: "Where does it hurt? And how can I help?"

In *Autopsy of a Suicidal Mind,* as well as in his other writings, Dr. Shneidman proves that he knows more about the psychological autopsy than anyone else in his field. Genuflecting to his peers in the field, Dr. Shneidman calls on distinguished colleagues, both those with whom he was closely associated at the beginning of his studies and other eminent experts in the field of suicide recovery, survival, and prevention, to give responses to the interviews with the family and friends of Arthur, the subject of this book. Old and wise, young and brilliant, ranging in age from 40 to 90, these commentators are colleagues and friends of Dr. Shneidman, and they have reflected and written essays about this tragic episode and the interviews of Arthur's family and friends. This collection of professional reflections is priceless and rare, and if words can heal—and in therapy words are the roots of healing in the shared exchange of ideas and emotions—there must be much healing that Arthur's mother and his family can gain from the insights of these experienced and emotionally generous comments.

From our first conversation on the phone, the professor and I talked as though we had known each other forever. There are, in Ed's home, the signs of his long life of study and contemplation—walls filled with art and books, whales of every description, a reflection of his lifelong study of Melville's writing and his great study of obsession and death, *Moby Dick.* We ate lunch in the garden as the March light poured onto us, filtered between the leaves of a tall, flowering jacaranda tree. Shneidman is now 86 years old, not in the best of health, and does not leave the house much. Of the two trips he made outside his home during 2002, one of them was to give a lecture at a nearby hospital, at which Arthur's mother presented Ed Shneidman with her son's 11-page suicide note.

Arthur and my son were both 33 when they took their lives. My son also left a suicide note, a 45-minute tape of his thoughts while dying; Arthur wrote his note over the course of a few days, leaving it at times, then coming back to fill in more of the pages with his feelings. At 33, both these talented, imaginative young men, beloved by their families and with histories of unhappiness and pain, died too young. I read *Autopsy of a Suicidal Mind,* and when Ed suggested that I write a foreword to the book, I immediately agreed. I was touched, and I of course identified with the pain of Arthur's mother and of his family. It seemed the least I could do for all of us who have suffered and for those who may want to think again, as they read this book, about the pain that comes to the survivors of any suicide.

In this book, the survivors of Arthur's suicide are interviewed and encouraged to talk about how they knew Arthur and what their feelings are about his life and death. This task helps the family and friends turn on the light and lets them see where they are and where they have been. The act of the interviews is an act of the removal of shame and the revelation that the family, as they say in the Alanon programs, "didn't cause it, couldn't cure it, and couldn't control it." The interviews put the suicide in perspective as the act of an individual, with individual motives, reasons, and, finally, responsibility. Each and every one of the family and friends did the best he or she could in the circumstances. That is all any of us can do.

Where are we to find the answers to the suicide of our loved one? Those of us who have lost friends or family need to talk about the terrible loss, the agony of questions, the anger and the hurt. We have to turn on the light, with each other and with strangers who have suffered the same fate. We look for permission to do this among a community that seldom understands this need, people who often will suggest that we "get on with it, forget it, move to the next phase of our lives." In other words, "stop talking about it."

But most of us *can't* move on. We have to talk it out and find a model for doing this, in therapy or in group counseling in which we share our stories with others who have suffered this terrible loss. We have to go through it all in order to "get out."

Dr. Shneidman's book shatters the secrets, opens the door to forgiveness of Arthur by his family, and to healing of each family member's own wounds. To be able to celebrate the life of our departed loved one and stop the crushing secrecy that can destroy us if we let it, we must go through the pain. *Autopsy of a Suicidal Mind* is a model of psychological autopsy that should help those who are bereft by a suicide to understand that the secrets are what often kill, and secrets can kill us if we don't let the light of truth and shared feelings enter our journey of grief.

For suicide to be transformed from taboo to understanding, we must seek to find why it is so forbidden a subject.

Arthur and my son Clark are gone. But their names and the stories of their lives can now be told. The light is on, and it must stay on. Only in the light can the taboo of suicide be healed, can the truth be sought, can the solace we survivors need be found. It is our own stories, our own words, our own journeys of healing that will bring the light of truth to shine on the dark taboo of suicide. Dr. Shneidman turns it on and lets it shine.

Thank you, Professor. We are indebted to you for ourselves and for the millions who went before, shrouded in secrets and silence. We no longer must walk in that dark place, for now we know that none of us is alone.

Judy Collins
New York City

PREFACE

The goal of this slim volume is quite simple: to provide readers with the inner details of one remarkable case study of a gifted young man who committed suicide, along with discussions of that case by some of the country's top suicide experts. It is hoped that the readers (some of whom will be anguished and puzzled survivors) might mine this extraordinary ore for their own nuggets of insight and solace.

Broadly speaking, one can discern two distinct approaches to the study of suicidal phenomena. We can call these approaches longitudinal and cross-sectional. Longitudinal studies are concerned with data over *time*—objective behavioral items such as a previous suicide attempt, divorce of the parents, failure in school, and so forth, particularly in early childhood. We call these prodromal clues or premonitory signs. The data are usually presented statistically, demographically, or epidemiologically. The nineteenth-century German philosopher Wilhelm Windelband called this view the *nomothetic* approach to knowledge.

On the other hand, the cross-sectional (or *idiographic*) approach is concerned with the more-or-less present: today, this month, now. What is going on (now)? How much do you hurt (now)? Its approach is more clinical, phrased in plain language, introspective, mentalistic.

Both approaches are needed to achieve maximum wisdom.

It should be obvious that this book is an intensive cross-sectional report of a single case. It is an idiographic study. I am pleased and proud to have done it. This book began by chance, unplanned and unexpected. A few years ago, I gave a lecture on suicide prevention in a nearby city. At the end of my presentation, a woman, comely and intense, approached me and gave me a copy of a suicide note written by her physician-lawyer son and asked me to read it and to share some of my thoughts with her. She soon sent me a list of names and telephone numbers of family members with whom I might talk. I am too old (in my mid-80s) to do things slowly. Within a few months, I had interviewed nine people—mother, father, brother, sister, pal, ex-wife, girlfriend, psychotherapist, and treating physician—and had sent sets of verbatim (edited) transcripts of those interviews to eight friends of mine, all world-class experts in suicidology, to comment on the deceased man, on his suicide, on what might have been done to save his life, and on the vast topic of suicide in general. This book is that psychological autopsy.

I humbly believe that, like every other detailed case study, this one has features that are unique and features that are ubiquitous. I believe that no reader, especially anyone whose life has been touched by this dire topic, can read it without gaining useful insights. In essence, this report is my special letter to that dear woman who shared her son's death, his suicide note, and his relatives and friends with me. In my concluding chapter, I have tried to set down my thoughts about this tragic case and about this merciless topic which has dominated my intellectual life

EDWIN S. SHNEIDMAN, Ph.D.
University of California, Los Angeles
September 2003

ACKNOWLEDGMENTS

No written book is a solo effort. I am happy publicly to give the identities of the people who helped me. Gabriele Jeffress was my indispensable and eager assistant, and Teresita Garcia was my life-extending health care helper.

My long-time agent, Regina Ryan, remains a stalwart friend and a joy in my life.

This is my second Oxford book—*The Suicidal Mind* (1996) was the first—and this is the second time I have had the good fortune to work with Joan Bossert. I have dubbed her Ms. Beaux Arts, or Beauxy for short, because that is what she is—one of the nicest people and one of the best editors in the world. Her assistant, Maura Roessner, was a right hand to both of us.

Of course, none of this would have happened without the active cooperation of the members of Arthur's family and the extraordinary efforts of the consultants who wrote their individual essays throwing light on the whole project.

CONTENTS

CONSULTANTS

NORMAN L. FARBEROW, Ph.D.
Former Codirector, Los Angeles
Suicide Prevention Center
Professor of Psychiatry (Psychology) Emeritus
University of Southern California

ROBERT E. LITMAN, M.D.
Former Chief Psychiatrist, Los Angeles
Suicide Prevention Center
Clinical Professor of Psychiatry
University of California at Los Angeles

JOHN T. MALTSBERGER, M.D.
Associate Clinical Professor of Psychiatry, Harvard University

RONALD W. MARIS, Ph.D.
Former Director, Suicide Center
Distinguished Professor Emeritus (Psychiatry, Sociology)
University of South Carolina

JEROME MOTTO, M.D.
Professor of Psychiatry Emeritus
University of California at San Francisco

M. DAVID RUDD, Ph.D.
Professor of Psychology, Baylor University
President, American Association of Suicidology

MORTON SILVERMAN, M.D.
Director, National Suicide Prevention
Technical Research Center
Editor, *Suicide and Life-Threatening Behavior*

AVERY D. WEISMAN, M.D.
Professor of Psychiatry Emeritus,
Harvard University
Former Director, Project Omega,
Massachusetts General Hospital

AUTOPSY OF
A SUICIDAL MIND

THE BEGINNING

Luckily for us, many important things in our lives happen serendipitously. Without a modicum of good luck, we would be rather unfortunate creatures. It was on a whim that I agreed to give a lecture (on suicide) at St. Pelagia's Hospital,[1] and it was fate that brought a grieving mother, Hannah Zukin, to hear me. At the end of my lecture, she came forward and said she had to talk to me for a few minutes. With some emotion, she told me of the recent suicide of her physician-lawyer son. She literally pressed into my hands a copy of an 11-page, handwritten suicide note. She asked me two questions. The first and most important was: Could I please give her some insights and some solace about the death of her boy? And the second question, no doubt prompted by her own clinical interest, was: How did I become involved in this dour field of human self-destruction?

I was taken by her immediately, and on impulse I said that I would try to help her. I believe that I am a man of my word, and I set about to do just that: to see what light might be shed on this tragic, enigmatic case. There and then she and I made arrangements to meet.

It's obvious that one of these two questions is easier to answer than the other, and so I turn to the second question first: how I became a suicidologist.

---

[1]St. Pelagia was a 15-year-old Christian girl who lived in the fourth century in ancient Turkish Antioch. When threatened with sexual assault by errant soldiers, she eluded them, and "in order to avoid outrage she threw herself to her death from a housetop roof" (Attwater, 1965). She is venerated by Catholics as a maiden martyr. One might say she is the patron saint of suicidology.

In 1949, when I was in my 30s, I was on the staff of the Veterans' Administration Neuropsychiatric Hospital in West Los Angeles. One day, the director of the hospital, Dr. James Rankin, called me into his office to ask me to write two letters of condolence for his signature to two newly created widows whose husbands, while wards of the hospital, had committed suicide. I felt that it would be useful to have as much information as possible, so I decided to go downtown to the coroner's office to look at the folders of these two men. The first folder contained something that I had never seen before: a genuine suicide note. The second did not. My curiosity was piqued, and I stayed in the coroner's vault all that day, looking at folders of hundreds of cases collected early in the twentieth century. I felt as though I were a Texas cowpoke stumbling home drunk who had fallen into a pool of pure undiluted oil. But something else happened at that very moment. Previously, when I was an undergraduate student at UCLA, I took courses in logic, in Descartes and John Stuart Mill. As a young student, I understood the Method of Difference—that you compare two groups, holding everything constant except one variable; then you can notice the subsequent differences between the two groups and can legitimately attribute those differences to the one item that you have introduced. So, in the coroner's office that fateful morning, John Stuart Mill's voice—it was he who wrote about the Method of Difference in his 1883 book *Essentials of Logic*—came into my head and said to me: You must not read these notes and be contaminated with their content because you will end up corroborating your preconceptions; rather, you should compare these with something that is like them but different. What to compare them with? Laundry lists? Love letters? Business correspondence? No. One should compare them with suicide notes written by *non*suicidal people. On the spot, I decided there could be elicited notes, simulated notes, suicide notes written by nonsuicidal persons.

I need to confess now—the statute of limitations has long since passed—that I "borrowed" some 721 suicide notes from the coroner's office. I then telephoned my friend and colleague, Dr. Norman Farberow, who subsequently became my intellectual partner for many years. He had just received his Ph.D. from UCLA and had completed a study on attempted suicides. Together we visited fraternal groups and labor unions and arranged for nonsuicidal Caucasian males—matched with Caucasian males who had committed suicide—to write the suicide notes that they would write if they were to take their own lives. We were then in a position to shuffle the suicide notes written by people who actually committed suicide (usually within the hour) and suicide notes written by people who clinically were not suicidal at all. It was a simple classic experiment, with "experimental" and "control" groups. Farberow and I spent 2 years analyzing the notes *blind*, that is, without knowing ourselves which notes were genuine and which were elicited.

In 1956, we wrote a five-page article for *Public Health Reports*. We received a small—$5,200—grant from the National Institute of Mental Health, and within 3 years we were the corecipients of a grant that turned out to be a 7-year award and totaled 1.5 million dollars. Contemporary suicidology had been born.

That is the story that, in one way or another, I shared with Mrs. Zukin, explaining why I was hooked on this lugubrious subject and how my fealty to this topic has never wavered over the past half century. More important, what I told her at St. Pelagia's Hospital that day was that I would try to generate information, hoping there would be insights and solace in that new material. That was the beginning of this project.

ABOUT SUICIDE NOTES

Collections of suicide notes have been available since the middle of the nineteenth century. Some writings about suicide notes typically have been anecdotal; others have been collections of notes without comment. As the reader already knows, my study of suicidal phenomena began in 1949 with my discovery of hundreds of suicide notes in the vaults of the Los Angeles County Coroner's office.

The scientific study of suicide—suicidology—may be said to have begun in 1957 with Shneidman and Farberow's publications of suicide notes (1957a, 1957b). Reproductions of suicide notes had been published since at least 1856 (Shneidman, 1979), but what was unique about Shneidman and Farberow's reports was the pioneer use of the "control" suicide note, that is, simulated suicide notes elicited from non-suicidal persons and then compared in "blind" studies with matched genuine suicide notes. Mill's Method of Difference—the heart of inductive science—was, for the first time, applied to the field of suicide.

At the very beginning, we believed (with excessive optimism) that, like Freud's notion about dreams being the royal road to the unconscious, suicide notes might prove to be the royal road to the understanding of suicidal phenomena. Reluctantly, after a decade or so of earnest efforts, I came to recognize that many notes are, in fact, bereft of the profound insights that we had hoped would be there. Now, it seems that we have come to rest somewhere in the middle, believing that, as a group, suicide notes are neither always psychodynamically rich nor psychodynamically barren, but rather, on occasion—when the note can be placed within the context of the known details of a life (of which that note is a penultimate part)—*then* words and phrases in the note can take on special meanings, bearing as they do a special freight within that context (Shneidman, 1973, 1980).

Our patient—call him Arthur—tells us at the very outset of *his* suicide note what the matter is. It is pain, psychological pain, what I call *psychache*. He hurts living in his own skin. He is wearing an unacceptable painful indwelling psychological catheter that is not adequately fitted, not adequately useful, and not adequately fulfilling. On the whole, he does not feel worthy. He is estranged, and he hurts beyond bearing.

He feels pessimistic about any future. Some time ago, early in his life, he formed a fixed idea, a flawed concept of what tolerable happiness might be, but his great tragedy was that he defined it in such a way that he could never attain it. It is present from the very beginning, in the very first few sentences. It is the pain, the enduring psychological pain that darkens his life. It is a pain that, in his psyche, is unbearable, intolerable, unendurable, and unacceptable. In his terms, it is better to stop the cacophony in his mind than to endure the unbearable noise.

Arthur's suicide note is not especially a cry for help. It is a testimonial and a plea for understanding. He tells us how badly he hurts; he asks us to understand his need for respite and peace of mind. In the beginning was the hurt; the rest is explication.

Perhaps I was drawn to this tragic case from the first words of Arthur's suicide note. In a sense, this case revolves around the note. It is in the note that the key questions are posed or implied. The note gives us some information: who's in and who's out, some of his key ambivalences, the flow of his thoughts and the restrictions of his reasoning, his flawed "therefores"; but it leaves unanswered basic questions of etiology which only systematic studies in psychology and other disciplines might address. In any event, in this round-robin of personal memories, this prolix suicide note is as close to a catamnestic report—that is, a patient history—from Arthur himself as we are able to get.

Arthur's note is like a giant tapeworm, with a small head at the beginning and an elongated, toxic tail. He says it all in the first paragraph, in the first five words: "All I do is suffer," and then, "Every moment is pain." The rest of his note is given to more or less pedestrian ramblings, instructions, and sentiments; the heart of the note is the cry at the beginning. There are some curious aspects to the note. We puzzle at the fact that there is no separate subnote addressed to his mother. Is this an inadvertent slip of his pen or a conspicuous omission? But again, the note is not about his love for others but about his all-consuming pain and his pressing need to find surcease and sanctuary from it, to stop the unbearable flow of consciousness that digs at his psyche like so many insulting poniards in his flesh.

I have chosen to reproduce the note (practically verbatim except for changes in names) not at this point in the book but, rather, at the end, in the appendix; I do this in order to get on with the business of the book rather than to stop the reader with this overwhelming, sometimes unbearable, sometimes pedestrian, sometimes poignant, sometimes even boring, document.

CONSULTATION BY
MORTON SILVERMAN, M.D.

Morton Silverman, M.D., is one of the more eminent of the second generation of American suicidologists. He was born in 1947 and is a product of the University of Pennsylvania and Northwestern University Medical School. Currently he is the director of the National Suicide Prevention Technical Resource Center based in Newton, Massachusetts. Previously he was chief of the Center for Prevention Research at the National Institute of Mental Health and Associate Administrator for Prevention in the Alcohol, Drug Abuse, and Mental Health Administration. His most recent positions were as associate professor of psychiatry, director of Student Counseling and Resource Service at the University of Chicago, and associate dean of students. Since 1996, he has been the editor in chief of Suicide and Life-Threatening Behavior, *the scientific journal of the American Association of Suicidology. He is one of the authors of the* Comprehensive Textbook of Suicidology.

This report might be called "The Man Who Knew Too Much." I approach the study of an individual's self-injurious death as a mystery that needs to be solved. Was it truly a suicide? Why was it a suicide? Does it "make sense" to me? Is it understandable? Often we are not left with much to study, other than the bare facts of the death and reports by police and medical examiners. In a relatively small minority of the cases a suicide note is left behind. So there is often much speculation about intent, motives, predisposing factors, and precipitating events.

The data regarding the death of Arthur are rich, thanks to the presence of a lengthy suicide note and interviews with four family members, two friends, a former wife, and two therapists. The psychological autopsy allows us an opportunity to see things from many different viewpoints, expressed by many different voices, and affords the investigator the luxury of "cutting and pasting" together details and perspectives to construct a cohesive picture. But in this case, do all these "extra" perspectives help us understand better what happened to Arthur (and why) beyond what he tells us in his own words?

Can we distill a narrative that "makes sense," that explains why he died as he did, or that puts to rest the immediate question that comes to mind: Why would a 30-something-year-old white male physician-lawyer kill himself when he allegedly has a supportive family, a close male friend, a loving girlfriend, a long-term psychotherapist, and a promising career?

The Suicide Note

The suicide note is a vehicle by which the decedent can have the last word. This mechanism allows the decedent to explain, to bring closure (or not), to assuage guilt, to dictate next steps, to control, to absolve, or to blame. I choose to focus mainly on Arthur's own words. What do we learn from Arthur's note? What is he trying to tell us? Do we need the interviews to illuminate and provide context to his narrative? I group some phrases that I found noteworthy.

1 *A need to control and direct:* "Please do not resuscitate me if alive when found. Please." "I want your happiness" (addressed to girlfriend). "[P]lease move on and make a marvelous life for yourself" (addressed to male friend). "You will survive without me" (addressed to male friend). "I need you to be happy that I'm out of pain" (addressed to sister).
2 *A plea for forgiveness:* "[R]emember me and be happy for me. Please be happy for me"; "I beg you to celebrate for me that I can be free of pain." "[P]lease understand that this is what I needed for me."
3 *An absolution:* "Those that tried to help me, including my therapist, should not feel that they failed"; "Don't feel you failed"; "No one should feel they failed."
4 *Ambivalence and uncertainty:* "I could not be saved I guess"; "I guess this was inevitable"; "Right now I am so torn."

5 *Poignant despair:* "[H]owever my periods of despair have sadly been there in much greater strength and preponderance." "Oh do I wish I was in a simple world where my only needs were food, shelter and clothing, and not some deep spiritual satisfaction." "I won't have to struggle with another day." "Understand that I was just suffering too much to bear anymore" (addressed to sister). "I will do it now. I have nothing left."

6 *Remorse and regret:* "I am sorry for leaving you" (addressed to male friend). "I want so badly to be back with my girlfriend. Why did I ever break up with her then?" "However, I feel that going back to her just may not be an option at this time." "I was not happy and felt there may be a woman out there that could just render me completely content with all of my life."

7 *Being a savior/being saved:* "She is all I feel can save me." "I guess I have always dreamt of myself as a savior being someone who would physically drag her off and force me into environments which were good for me and lead me to pleasures in my life." "If there is anything above when we are gone, then I will be smiling at you as a close friend when I see you happy in your life. Marry and raise a family" (addressed to girlfriend).

8 *Altruism:* "If I go this evening, then I go to spare her more unnecessary pain and to avoid our inevitable cycle of torture."

9 *Lack of pleasure:* "How long can one go without pleasure?" "[A]nd this has taken a great toll on me without anything giving me pleasure in life."

10 *Self-criticism:* "It is the last years that I have managed to slowly ruin my life." "I can't hold it together long enough." "[E]ven if I have been bad at keeping in touch." "I can't handle pressure." "I lived in isolation. I did not adjust to the school." "Somehow I made it through that period." "They [the problems] are within me." "My life is a tragedy, but it is one that I unfortunately cannot overcome."

Some Curious Contradictions

Arthur clearly states that he wants his organs donated but wants no autopsy done. "NO AUTOPSY. Leave my body alone"; but later he says, "Please DONATE MY ORGANS if possible." As a physician, he should know that all suicides and almost all deaths by overdose are investigated by the office of the medical examiner and necessitate an autopsy. He knew his organs would die along with his brain, so he should have known that by the time his body was discovered, most of his organs (maybe except for his corneas and skin) would not be acceptable for transplantation. He poisoned his brain. Why would he think that his organs would not be poisoned as well?

Some of his most poignant writing is evident in his 8:00 A.M. note. This note was being written by a man who was throwing up from a serious suicide attempt by overdose. So, what does he do? He plans to try again that night—not in the upcoming hours, because he has a plan to meet with his male friend in the morning and with his father for their usual Sunday lunch. I find it curious that he survives a "failed attempt," is determined to try again, but must first reconnect with the world he is determined to leave, all the time explaining in more written detail his rationale for dying.

Here is a man who tells us repeatedly that he is "a person who doesn't care about anything," yet he proceeds to write an extensive suicide note documenting his despair, while demonstrating how much he truly cares about his girlfriend, male friend, brother, and sister, whom he specifically addresses individually.

His ambivalence is pervasive, both in his note and in his behavior over the weekend. As a physician, he had clear knowledge about efficient and effective means to end his life. He would also have access to multiple medications that could be lethal. The fact that he chose to overdose with lithium and a synthetic narcotic analgesic and that he did not die on his first attempt on that Friday night speaks to a certain degree of ambivalence.

The note supports a picture of a man who is self-centered, self-critical, exhausted with struggling not to feel isolated, and experiencing a range of emotions, including ambivalence, regret, despair, and fear. He is in psychological pain, with little perception of the meaning of relationships with significant others in his life. What additional information does the psychological autopsy method provide? For one, we learn much more about his weekend activities. He called his girlfriend on Friday night and threatened suicide if she didn't come back to him—a "cry for help." Yet, his girlfriend reports that he had done this many times before. Were the meetings with his male friend on Sunday morning and his father at noon on Sunday another "cry for help" or a "failed attempt" to be rescued? Interestingly, he doesn't mention these "intervening" weekend events in his note. Arthur says his serious high school suicide attempt was not a cry for help, because he was truly intent on dying; yet he "aborted" it himself. Were the prolonged process of dying, his weekend activities, and the extensive notes communication about his lifelong despair and his ambivalence about dying? And maybe even his wish to be rescued individually by three of the most important people in his life?

Going by the Numbers

It is easy to categorically state that Arthur had a significant number of risk factors that, in combination, pushed him toward suicide. Some of these risk factors are: history of being bullied at school (and also admittedly by his brother); history of a learning disability, diagnosed in college ("auditory discriminatory problem"); poor school performance until high school; clear cognitive, physical, and psychosocial developmental delays (reading, speech, coordination); severe behavioral tantrums at home and at school (up to ages 10–12); parental divorce at age 10; rigid maternal nurturing; history of at least one suicide attempt; history of psychiatric inpatient hospitalization; history of early onset of psychopathology (with psychotherapy from ages 7–15); history of running away from school and from home; history of food phobias (indicative of possible irrational childhood fears); thumb sucking until age 9; history of poor socialization in childhood and early adolescence; his own marital discord, leading to divorce (after 3 years); and a history of family psychopathology (mother and brother with depressive episodes, maternal grandmother on antidepressants). Although the risk factors are certainly there, do they explain his suicide? Did his protective factors "neutralize" some of these negative risk factors? Were there intervening variables or precipitating events that became heightened as a result of this profile?

Nature versus Nurture

This case illustrates the interplay and tension in a mind-versus-brain approach to understanding self-destructive behavior. There is little doubt that Arthur had some type of neurological delays or disruptions in early infancy and childhood (up to age 12), as exemplified by severe temper tantrums, running away from home and school, disruptions in the classroom, biting his mother, swinging a baseball bat in the home, and wildly running through the home. His mother described him as dysphoric and anhedonic.

It is unclear how these behavioral problems and poor ability to relate to others interfered with the development of a nurturing relationship between Arthur and his mother. His mother alludes to her own bouts of depression and to feeling overwhelmed as a mother. One has to wonder if she might have been subclinically depressed and "outmatched" by a "difficult child." She describes Arthur as frustrated, frightened, angry, and full of rage. This presentation clearly made his brother seem "supernormal" as they grew up in close proximity to each other. Whatever the neurological "insults" and "storms" were, they seemed not to have caused permanent cognitive deficits, as evidenced by Arthur's academic successes. However, these temper tantrums may have left deficits in his emotional equilibrium, sense of self, and ability to soothe himself.

The perception of abandonment and dissolution of the family structure (and holding environment) following his parents' divorce at age 10 only added to Arthur's difficulties as a child. He apparently blamed his mother for the divorce. However, at some level, could he keep from blaming himself for contributing to the divorce? According to his psychotherapist, his parents' divorce was contentious, and Arthur might have been unable to tolerate his own resultant fear of abandonment and disappointments. His basic sense of trust was assaulted and further complicated by the parents' need to maintain "family secrets," particularly those relating to his own adolescent suicide attempt and subsequent hospitalization.

We will never know whether a change in medications might have helped. What is clear is that Arthur discontinued his antidepressants 6 months before his death and refused further chemotherapy or electroconvulsive therapy. He had not been in psychotherapy for 2 1/2 years, and, despite his prior behavior, he apparently did not see the need to reengage with his long-term psychotherapist. He was said to be very sensitive to shame. Yet is this the expected behavior of a trained physician who knew he was prone to depression and feared the onset of another depressive episode?

A Developmental Perspective

This man seems to have been on a mission—a search—to find an identity, peace of mind, emotional stability, a sense of predictability, and security. Every time he approached it, it eluded him for one reason or another. The high school incident that led to his first suicide attempt was probably due to his realization that the wonderful weekend experience was fleeting and elusive and that he didn't have the wherewithal to ensure that he could create and maintain such good feelings by himself. He knew he needed supports, and they weren't there for him at that time. He went to medical school to identify with his dad—to be financially successful and to be a family man. He married at age 24.

When medical school no longer was a challenge, or no longer provided him with needed sustenance, he went to law school. Once there, he doubted that he deserved to be there. His ex-wife says that Arthur was very judgmental and harsh—toward himself and toward others. If he wasn't the best, he felt that he was nothing at all. Although nobody could live up to his standards, inside he felt like a fraud. His psychotherapist reports that a major therapeutic triumph occurred when Arthur was able to accept that he might not be the best Scrabble player in town—and that that was okay.

While in medical school, after 3 years of a troubled marriage, he got divorced and became depressed. This was the point at which he began psychopharmacological treatment with a psychiatrist, who observed that he was acutely suicidal. His mother says that it was in medical school that Arthur made a second suicide attempt. He had found another woman to love, but every time they seemed to get close, he ran away (over and over again). Intimacy and vulnerability seemed to scare him. He constantly was searching for people, institutional frameworks, and careers to provide him with the "fix" for his pleasureless world. His girlfriend reports that he wasn't happy with life. He couldn't make the sadness go away, and he couldn't find happiness.

It remains unclear to me whether he sought a medical education to better understand the etiology, pathogenesis, treatment, management, and prognosis of his struggles with himself. He probably became a physician to achieve a sense of authority, mastery, and control. He may have seen the "white coat" as a means to resolve his jealousies, competitive drive, and sense of low self-esteem. He was already struggling with chronic feelings of self-doubt (whether he got into medical school on his own merits) and ambivalence (Is a career in medicine right for me?). Are these the "life's struggles" that he refers to in his suicide note?

A Psychiatric Perspective

It seems that he was unable to store all the loving, caring, and support that were directed at him for an emotional "rainy day." Arthur seemed to lack any psychic reserve. His emotional well was always empty, and he lurched from one fleeting pleasurable episode to another. However, no relationship, no event, and no professional identity lasted very long or long enough. His ex-wife reports that Arthur's times of utmost despair came immediately after happy times. Was he aware of the extent to which he couldn't store, retrieve, or generate good feelings? Again, perhaps the sequelae of a neurological insult at an early age? That remains unknown.

Of note is that he died on a Sunday night—after a weekend of struggling with his emptiness, fears of failure, and sense of abandonment (again reinforced by his girlfriend's refusal to restart their relationship yet another time). In fact, his girlfriend went out of town on Saturday morning. Perhaps he now physically and emotionally perceived her as out of reach. On Friday night he had called her and begged for her to come back to him, all the while threatening to kill himself if she refused. Interestingly, his ex-wife reports a similar pattern: After they divorced, he ardently pursued her in an attempt to reunite.

Facing another week of challenges to his emotions, his credibility, his medical knowledge, his equilibrium, his cohesiveness, and his fragile identity probably was too much for him—especially when he sensed the insidious onset of symptoms similar to those of his prior bouts with depression. At the age of 28, Arthur had told his psychiatrist that if he had another depression, he would kill himself.

Another possible explanation is that the depressive episode had already begun and that the illness already was interfering with his cognitive and emotional stability and processing ability. His psychiatrist observes that Arthur saw a return of a depression as a reminder of his imperfection. He may have had a prescient sense that he was already on that trajectory, and the illness itself prevented him from clearly thinking of alternatives.

Arthur already had experienced an inpatient psychiatric hospitalization, psychotherapy, medication, medical school, law school, a marriage, a girlfriend, and a long-term buddy relationship. He had tried living with a woman (his ex-wife), with his brother, and then with his best friend. He compartmentalized his life into small, manageable units. He was restless emotionally and intellectually. His male friend reports that he had difficulty asking for help. His ex-wife reports that he never was satisfied. He was said to be bored and pessimistic and to feel that life had no meaning. He felt terribly alone, even when he was in a marriage. His ex-wife says that he would withdraw and not communicate for days at a time. Can you imagine how he felt when he was all alone in his apartment and in constant fear of abandonment? Was his death preventable?

The interviewees indicate that Arthur was likeable, attractive, good-natured, and funny. He was not psychotic or wildly unpredictable as an adult. One can't help but identify with some of his difficulties. Who can't relate to his adolescent struggles and frustrations? Some of his moments of despair are tangible and totally understandable.

How could anyone have saved Arthur? Possibly by offering him unconditional empathy and understanding. Possibly by acknowledging and respecting his pain and daily struggles. Possibly by convincing him that there was potential hope to learn how to accept love, to give love, to sustain himself from day to day, to laugh at himself, to ask for help without feeling helpless, to ask for and accept empathy and understanding, and to accept being a patient. I would not convey that I could take away his pain or his susceptibility to repetitive depressive episodes nor that I could relieve him of his pervasive negative views—only that I would want to work with him to contain them and control them. His psychiatrist in medical school described him as having a chronic psychiatric malignancy. With his permission, I would have tried to engage his girlfriend in couples therapy and his family in family therapy. Group therapy might have offered him a chance to see that others suffer as well and struggle to stay alive. Another attempt at medications was indicated. Electroconvulsive therapy (ECT) might have been of great help and provided relief.

Yet had he not already been protected from a premature death? He was sustained for many years by a dedicated psychotherapist and a perceptive psychiatrist, who offered him hope (through psychotherapy and medication) and provided caring and respect. He lived for thirteen years beyond his first serious suicide attempt (which required hospitalization). He reports that he never truly gave up the thought or intent to die. My sense is that right up until the end he wanted to be saved but didn't know how to save himself without asking for help—which, ironically, he may have been too ashamed to ask for. He also desperately wanted to be understood and accepted. Could he have been saved? Without his willingness to accept help and be labeled as a patient, I believe the long-term prognosis was poor.

A Final Note

What I find most tragic about this case is that here we have a very bright young man, well educated and well trained in two demanding professions, who had available to him multiple resources, as well as much knowledge about treatment modalities and alternatives. That, in the end, he chose to reject options available to him (such as inpatient or outpatient ECT, inpatient psychiatric treatment, outpatient psychiatric treatment, and medical consultation about alternative approaches to chemotherapy) is a tragedy. This is a case of a young man searching for authenticity, identity, and individuation. Every time he entered into situations that allowed him a taste of these things, they weren't sustainable—either due to circumstances (the high school weekend) or to his inability to adjust to them (his marriage, a long-term commitment to his girlfriend).

What I conclude is that this man could not and would not allow himself to enter into another depressive episode, because he was intensely afraid of the psychological pain associated with it. He knew he had no psychic reserves to draw on. I believe that, because he was already struggling with a constant feeling of emotional emptiness and loneliness, the addition of an impending major depressive episode would overwhelm his abilities to function as a physician-lawyer, friend, son, sibling, and lover. He perceived that his fragile and vulnerable hold on self-identity could not withstand another bout of depression, with its known devastating effects on his sense of control, on his ability to access the full range of his mental and emotional facilities, and on his sense of safety, stability, and security.

Nothing completely satisfied him or sustained him for long periods of time. He knew he lived a fragile and tenuous existence, held together by daily routines and sometimes by well-meaning but unsustainable relationships with concerned family and friends. He knew this house of cards was makeshift at best and unpredictable at worst. He knew the pain he endured daily and feared the pain that was coming. He was too "smart" for his own good. And therein lay the ultimate tragedy, the ultimate enigma, and the ultimate paradox.

INTERVIEW WITH
THE MOTHER

Without exception, the interviews with each of the seven family members and two professionals went well. We had good rapport and mutual respect. All nine interviews were done within one 6-month period, all within a few months of Arthur's death. Although an established protocol exists for conducting a psychological autopsy, with these nine special people I certainly did not have a checklist of questions. Common sense (and common courtesy) dictated the flow of talk. In each case, my interactions were guided by four pinpoints of focus: (1) What sort of person was he? (Tell me about Arthur); (2) What went into his suicide? (Tell me your understanding of why he killed himself); (3) What are your ideas about suicide in general? (Tell me your notions of human self-destruction); and (4) What do you think might have been done to prevent his death? (Could his life have been saved and how might that have been done?)

Here are verbatim excerpts from the interview with Arthur's mother—reprinted by permission.

ESS: *Please tell me what happened.*
MOM: Where do you want me to start?
ESS: *It doesn't matter.*
MOM: I'll tell you from when he was a child. Arthur was a very sweet little boy, but by two years old he was having horrible tantrums, temper tantrums. He didn't speak, but he would scream and yell and flail and he was very difficult. And he has a twenty-two-month-older brother who was very rambunctious. And I always called Arthur "my little girl" because as an infant he was always fairly

quiet but always inquisitive but quiet, and my other son is very active. Arthur was very subdued except that he had horrible temper tantrums. In kindergarten everybody thought he was a very sweet little boy because he had a very sweet demeanor but he could go very wild and crazy and one time in kindergarten he got so upset he knocked the teacher's glasses off. She was totally flabbergasted and she called me, of course. I told her that he had many temper tantrums at home also but that he was usually able to contain them at other places.

ESS: *Was there any intimation of what set him off?*

MOM: The least provocation set him off. He way overreacted to things and, as the years go by, I realize that there was very much overreaction to anything that upset him in any way. He wasn't very articulate. He didn't talk. He was not articulate as a young child. He didn't speak really until he was almost three, and then it was in sentences. But he was always competing with his brother, who was articulate at twelve or thirteen months old and sort of ran the household. So Arthur was always competing with him, and he didn't speak a lot. He was creative, he was busy with his hands, he did models and he did buildings and he crawled on the floor and explored electrical outlets. But he was always in competition with his brother, and he didn't read very well until he was seven or eight years old. And he was always frustrated, he had a very frustrating school experience. By the third grade he was absolutely horrible, he was just having such a horrible time, he started having therapy from that time on, seeing a psychotherapist twice a week, and the school was so frustrating for him. It is so painful to remember all this. He couldn't do his homework, he couldn't do anything, so we decided, the principal with whom we were all good friends, the principal and the teachers, that he would not have any extra homework from the third grade. The teachers wanted to send him home early and we said, no, we were paying a lot of money so we wanted him to go the full day. Later on we recognized he had a learning disability. A neighbor who was a speech therapist kept telling me but I did not listen to her. Arthur found out in college that he had an auditory discriminatory problem, that he couldn't hear and process material, and he learned by reading, not by hearing. He graduated Phi Beta Kappa from university, made top honors in medical school and law school, so he obviously was smart. He knew what was going on, but as a young kid we didn't know he had this learning problem.

ESS: *So you are describing a sensitive, almost neurologically sensitive, youngster.*

MOM: And in fact he went to law school after he went to medical school. His father is a physician, so he thought that he should do that. He said all through college he used to bring the crossword puzzle and read the newspaper in all of his classes because the information didn't process through his brain when he heard a lecture. After hearing the lecture, he would then go read, and that was how he learned, and he learned how to compensate for that, obviously, and did very well in his way of compensating. But as a little child, we weren't aware he had this learning problem.

ESS: *And how did he seem?*

MOM: He was brazen in a lot of ways; he was obstinate. He seemed like a frightened child, but he acted out in a fearless way.

ESS: *Tell me what your clues were that he seemed like a frightened child.*

MOM: His whole demeanor, [his defense is so loud] that it felt like he was warding off his fears in an angry way. He was frustrated that he couldn't learn. And at night, the two boys shared a room, his brother would read in bed and Arthur, twenty-two months younger, would not be reading; the brother would be eight or nine and Arthur would be seven and he couldn't really read or enjoy it and he would say to his older brother, I bet you're just turning the pages. He was more angry that he couldn't get it.

ESS: *So that on top of this there is an intense rivalry.*

MOM: Very intense. Physically, too. Arthur was very slender and skinny and his brother was bigger and very athletic.

ESS: *Can you tell me more about the content of his fears?*

MOM: I'm not sure. He was afraid more of himself somehow, I don't know how to put it.

ESS: *What aspects of himself?*

MOM: His inability to be what he thought was expected of him. Academically he had a huge frustration. I realize in our home there must have been a great emphasis on academics. I didn't think that I pushed it, but because his brother was so advanced, it was just there in the household, and I think it was a constant source of frustration to Arthur. So I think it was more a sense of frustration than fear.

And then, physically, his brother always overpowered Arthur physically and took advantage of him in play. When the brother took the LSAT—he is now in law school—he scored in the 99th percentile. He is very bright. His grades go up and down, he has As and Fs. He is very brilliant. Arthur was also, but we didn't recognize it. Arthur's mind was very scientific and different. When Arthur graduated Phi Beta Kappa, we weren't on good terms at that time, and his father found out about it. He didn't want anybody to know. Apparently there was a dinner inducting the new Phi Beta Kappas and somehow his father found out, and his father and his then wife were driving there, and I had found out just that day; and I called Arthur, and he was in the library. His friends answered the phone, and finally I got ahold of him, and he said you better don't come up here I do not want you there. And I turned around and went home. We were divorced since Arthur was ten, and he told me he didn't even want his father to come, but he knew his father was paying for school and so he felt somehow obligated that his father had to come, but he didn't like to tell anybody about his achievements. He was punishing me.

ESS: *For?*

MOM: I didn't know what. He was always angry at me, always angry. He took all his anger out on me, all of it. He didn't hate me. His girlfriend, his wife, all told me how much he loved me, but somehow he wouldn't let me know it.

ESS: *What was he angry at you about?*

MOM: I think all of his frustrations.

ESS: *Was the divorce your fault in his mind?*

MOM: I think he thought that but not really as a young child. Nobody knew I did want the divorce, but it wasn't my fault. I wanted the divorce. I wanted my husband to leave.

ESS: *What was the divorce about?*

MOM: I didn't realize until much later. In the beginning I said I was bored and felt unsupported by my husband; and I have come to realize in my own mind that there was a lack of connection between us. I just didn't feel like husband and wife. I was responsible for my four children; they were very difficult children. I made all the decisions; I was not working, of course, and I took them everywhere, always running, running, running; doing everything with the children. Two children going to psychotherapy twice a week, that's four different psychotherapy appointments four days a week, you know; and then one daughter, who is three years younger than Arthur, and her activities, and the other daughter six years younger. I just felt that the children were so difficult, the boys were so difficult, and I felt like my ex-husband didn't support me. And, in fact, he and I have talked about it, and he said he didn't support me. He was mad at how I was raising the children; he felt I was too strict because I said they had to have a bedtime. He didn't think children needed a bedtime; he grew up without a bedtime, jumping on the furniture. So I was way too strict, he said; so he didn't agree with how I was raising the children; we recently had this discussion. Now we're going out together again, just spending a lot of time together. His divorce will be final in a couple of weeks. As a result of Arthur's death, he was having a miserable marriage, and I think this just brought things to a head. He has told me how much he has loved me all these years and how wrong our divorce was and how devoted he was to me and that he was never as devoted or dedicated to his second wife; that she never meant the same that I meant to him.

ESS: *Permit me to change the topic. How much do you see in Arthur the push of genes, genetics, temperament, early disposition?*

MOM: I myself have a tendency to depression, as does my mother. My mother is taking antidepressants. Well, I was going to say at that point I was depressed, I was miserable in this situation, and then after I got divorced I was really depressed. I told my ex-husband there were times that I thought I was suicidal because I was over-whelmed with the care of four children who were just crushing my life.

ESS: *Have you attempted suicide in your life?*

MOM: No, and I never would because of my children. I thought of it but I never would. I understand how he could have done it.

ESS: *Tell me who you are.*

MOM: I was a very shy, unconfident person until I got married, and then somehow that gave me a lot of security and a lot of confidence. All of a sudden I became my own person.

ESS: *Did you have siblings?*

MOM: I have a sister. She is younger than I, and we don't have a very close relationship. I love her, but we're not good friends. She is always jealous.

ESS: *How much of a topic is Arthur's death in your life and in your family today?*

MOM: I'd talk about it, if it were up to me, constantly, if it were up to me [tearful]. My mother, who is still alive, I talk to her about it constantly. I talk to my mother, my sister somewhat I talk about it, I feel comfortable. With my extended family, they don't like to hear it. They tell me to get on with my life and to concentrate on the other children.

ESS: *Would they be pleased to hear, if this occurs, that you are remarrying?*

MOM: Everybody would. And the one who would have been most pleased would have been Arthur, because he was devastated by the divorce; it shook him more than the other three children.

ESS: *I've asked this before, did he blame you for that?*

MOM: I don't know, I think he probably did, but he didn't know that it was my fault. I guess he did blame me. But he was angry at me before the divorce. The divorce didn't cause his problem, it exacerbated it. He was having tantrums every day, horrible tantrums; he would run through the house and take a baseball bat and swing a baseball bat around the house. I would have to contain him and confine him. I would sit on him and I would hold his arms. And he'd bite my hair or bite my arms and I'd cry.

ESS: *What could he be saying when he did this?*

MOM: I don't know, I don't remember. He was just crying, screaming, "Leave me alone, leave me alone," and I used to call his psychologist and be on the phone with the psychologist at the time and he'd say, "You're doing the right thing, just contain him, just contain him." I wasn't trying to hurt him, just trying to stop him. His sisters would be sleeping, he'd run in and jump on their beds and wake them up. Sometimes during the day he would be running through the house. I remember during the day when he would get so crazy I would tell [his sister] "Go to"—her best friend lived across the street—I would say, "maybe you should go play with your best friend, Arthur is having a really bad time right now." For thirty years I've tried to raise him to be a vital human being, and it was a struggle the whole time, and it was all on me. There was no one else who really participated. I tried. I knew he was depressed. Later, I used to call him, and he wouldn't accept my phone calls. I'd leave messages: "Are you taking your medication, how are you doing, how are you doing?" He wouldn't see me very often. He saw his father every week for breakfast; every Sunday they met. When he wanted to see his father, he would call his father, and they'd always meet at a restaurant on the other side of town. And it was very superficial. Arthur never said anything, except, about a month before he died, he told his father that he hated everything, that everything was bad; he hated his school, he hated girls, he hated everything. And his father said, "Just put a smile on your face and pretend it's okay." If Arthur would have told me that, I would have been terrified, but he wouldn't dare tell me that.

ESS: *It doesn't mean that he's going to commit suicide; but it means that there will be perturbation in his life, that this is part of his life, he seems built that way.*

MOM: I do want people to understand that he was a special person who lived a very tormented life, as I did as a result, trying just to take care of him, and it drove the whole family crazy; and his older brother, too, has his own problems, between the two of them, but I was just a mess for thirty years, trying to take care of him. It destroyed my life, it was my life, I couldn't do anything else but take care of my children. I did, and I went back to school and got my Master's after I got divorced. I have to live beyond that. That doesn't mean that I can't love and get love.

THE IDEA OF A
PSYCHOLOGICAL AUTOPSY

At my first meeting with Arthur's mother, she presented to me a typed list of names and telephone numbers of other relatives, which also included Arthur's long-term psychotherapist and the physician who attended him toward the end. She asked me if I would be interested in talking with these other people. Without knowing it, she was suggesting a psychological autopsy of Arthur's enigmatic death.

The psychological autopsy procedure was developed at the Los Angeles Suicide Prevention Center (SPC) during the 1960s, specifically at the request of Theodore J. Curphey, M.D., then chief medical examiner and coroner of Los Angeles County. The primary purpose of the psychological autopsy is quite simple: to assist the coroner in making decisions for the death certificate as to the most appropriate *mode* of death—the modes of death are natural, accident, suicide, and homicide (the so-called NASH categories)—in cases in which the mode of death, at first look, seems equivocal or uncertain. (This uncertainty usually devolves between accident and suicide.) The procedure was created and conducted by the behavioral scientists (psychiatrists, psychologists, and social workers) of the staff of the SPC. The procedure is done by interviewing people relevant to the task; namely, people who knew the deceased—spouse, grown children, relatives, employers, associates, lovers, and others. The goal is to obtain information which might throw light on the *intention* of the decedent vis-à-vis his or her own death; that is, if he or she wanted death to occur, then it was suicide, but if he or she would have been surprised by death, then it was an accident. This procedure (about which there were many questions at the beginning) also serves to assuage some of the feelings of guilt and shame of the survivors and has a general therapeutic mental health effect in the community.

In some few cases, the psychological autopsy is used even though the mode of death is unequivocal; specifically, in cases in which death is clearly suicidal (with suicide notes). In these few cases, the goal of the procedure is to help understand the *why* of the suicidal death. That is the kind of psychological autopsy that is being done in this case. The mode is (regrettably) crystal clear, but the reasons are murky, and the event begs for some possible further clarification. The psychological autopsy has been used in civil suits and even in a court martial, with dramatic effectiveness (Shneidman, 1993). It has caught on.[1]

In 1950, Akira Kurosawa, the fabled Japanese filmmaker, directed *Rashomon*, one of the classic motion pictures of all time. It is a story of an incident in a forest in medieval Japan in which "something" happens between an errant bandit (played brilliantly by Toshiro Mifune) and a beautiful young Japanese noblewoman. There are other participants in this drama: the woman's husband, a woodcutter, and, of course, the girl herself and the bandit. The film begs the question, What *really* happened in the forest that fateful afternoon? The film is enduring because it is a philosophical piece, specifically an epistemological exercise. What is Truth? Whose point of view are we to believe? Does any of them tell the total story? What is the reliability of witnesses to a fateful event? and so forth. These questions (and others) are the background of this present psychological autopsy in which the mode of death—suicide—is clear but in which the questions surrounding the event draw us into a larger (epistemological, psychological, psychiatric) discussion.

This report concerns a 33-year-old male Caucasian who was both a physician and an attorney and who committed suicide by means of a drug overdose. His parents are nonobservant Jews of central European descent. He killed himself in a large metropolitan area in the United States in the early years of the twenty-first century.

---

[1]From the beginning I believed in the psychological autopsy—which I had the pleasure of naming—based as it was on the commonsense principle that additional relevant information is always helpful in any intellectual enterprise. The idea of the psychological autopsy has caught on. In a recent publication, Jie Zhang et al. (2002) indicate that in the decade between 1990 and 2001 there were over 120 publications, worldwide, on the psychological autopsy—in the United States, United Kingdom, Finland, Japan, Malaysia, India, and other countries.

Verbatim data from 10 sources are reported. The first source is excerpts from the decedent's handwritten suicide note; the other nine are verbatim excerpts from interviews that I conducted with the following persons: (1) Arthur's mother; (2) his father; (3) his older brother; (4) his younger sister; (5) his best friend; (6) his former wife; (7) his current girlfriend; (8) his long-term psychotherapist; and (9) the physician who treated him.

Eight eminent suicidologists, acting as independent discussants, have commented on these psychological autopsy data. They have addressed the tantalizing questions of the possible etiologies of Arthur's suicidal death and have shared their reflections as to what, if anything, might have been done to save his life.

Further information on the psychological autopsy can be found in Curphey (1961); Litman, Curphey, Shneidman, Farberow, and Tabachnick (1963); Shneidman (1977); and Weisman (1974).

INTERVIEW WITH
THE FATHER

ESS: *To put it formally, you are the decedent's father. Please tell me briefly who you are, and then tell me about Arthur.*

DAD: I am Arthur's father. I'm a physician. I've always been a family man, very much involved in my children's life and concerned with them and proud of them; and Arthur gave me much delight over the years. To me he was a wonderful, loving son. I'm divorced from his mother for many years, since he was ten years old. His older brother was twelve and his sisters were seven and three. We had joint custody with the children, and the kids would be with me for one week and with their mother for one week. Until the time of the divorce, from the time Arthur was born, I would consider myself to have been an involved father. I used to read him stories and play games with him and help him with his homework. We were in Indian Guides together, and we would do projects together in the house. He had very difficult years of growing up while we were married; he went into therapy when he was approximately seven years old and used to have—I'd call them tantrums. He didn't seem to have a good image of himself; whereas his older brother was much more academic and much more athletic, Arthur developed very slowly in those areas. At twelve he was going to therapy, and he was acting out really very physically, fighting with his brother, running out of the house, breaking things, and doing very poorly academically in school. Then, when he was about twelve, there seemed to be sort of a metamorphosis, a whole change in him, where he did a project on Hannibal crossing the Alps. He made the little figures, he made the mountain, he wrote a short story on this large project; it was a three-dimensional project. And he got an A+, you know, A on effort, A on presentation, A on materials, and all of a sudden Arthur started to become very good academically. He also had orthodontics done; he had been sucking his thumbs till he was nine years old, and with the braces he started to be more attractive. His whole image, physically and mentally; he started doing so well with friends, with teachers. And no more acting out. Perhaps, looking back, it was all sublimated, all internalized, all this pain that he was going through. Before that there was a lot of this acting out, where he would throw things or fight with his mother or his brother, not much with me. We were told by the therapist during those years that we should just hold him. Just protect him so he wouldn't hurt himself or others when he was so agitated. He had very good friends during those early years as well. He had a best friend who lived next door since they were born; and they played almost every day, did models together, played other games together; they eventually even went to camp together when they were ten. In Indian Guides, when he was about six—I remember that very clearly—he had just started, and we were on a retreat for the weekend, and he had climbed up a tree with another kid, and I heard that kid say to him, "Arthur, we'll be friends forever." He had a certain thing in his personality that people really liked to be with him. And of course this extended all the way into his adult years, where Arthur, on the surface, was not only attractive physically, and intellectually very aware and alert, but there was some magnetism in his personality that people loved to be with him. I was certainly left out of the loop in understanding the severity of his problems. I knew that he tried to commit suicide when he was around fourteen; he had been away for a camp retreat. He was going to a religious high school at that time, which is a supplemental school; a few days during the week he'd go there for two hours and then the retreats up to a camp up in the mountains. And Arthur had gone on this encampment; and again, I heard all this afterwards, shortly after Arthur died, that Arthur had had such a wonderful time. He put that in his letters at one time when he was attempting suicide but did not, a few years before this actual horrible event. That he had gone to camp and apparently he had such a wonderful time, he came back and in his mind felt that it couldn't be duplicated; he was going back into the rut of being in school and not really feeling good, and so he should leave life on this high, whatever that means. And that's when he took an excessive dose of Tylenol, but he was with his mother that night; a Sunday night, apparently, after the weekend, and then we were told what he had done, and she took him to the hospital. And thank God he survived; but after that neither I nor his mother were told: be alert, be aware, do something; he is very prone to doing this again; this is a bad sign for the future—we were not made aware of anything.

ESS: *He was in therapy at that time?*

DAD: I don't know the year he stopped, but definitely from age five to about fifteen. We sent him and his brother to therapists all through the years, whatever the cost. Obviously, it didn't work, and we feel very angry, very disappointed. And then, of course, Arthur seemed to have wonderful years after this attempted suicide. He graduated high school way high up, academically, with girlfriends, boyfriends; he went on a trip abroad when he was sixteen. He was part of the "in group." Everyone loved him, and he appeared so happy. I visited him while he was in Europe and spent a weekend with him with relatives. They all adored him. Then, after high school, he decided he wanted to be a physician like his dad, like me. He had no pressure from me there. I said do whatever you want. He was debating between law and medicine. And because I enjoyed the field all these years, 30-plus years now, he apparently felt that it probably would be a good choice. Turned out to be the wrong choice. After medicine, he changed over to law, but he didn't hold me responsible because, and this was one of the smartest things I ever did, I never said: be a physician. I said do what you want; I can only say that I've been having a good time in this field.

ESS: *In what ways was it wrong?*

DAD: He said he liked the academics so much more. And he got in immediately into medical school. And in law school he was outstanding, he was going to clerk for a Supreme Court justice, and all kinds of other things. So he wasn't leaving out of weakness, only emotionally he didn't want that. He, I think, wanted the excitement of a group, of a feel, and evidently this was not being transmitted to him. And in law he thought he would get more, and he did. From my understanding, law was wonderful for him, and he excelled.

ESS: *Of belonging to a larger group?*

DAD: Well, our family; I was raised by a father with high ideals and high aspirations. I've always been involved in the community with ideals, aspirations, challenges, high expectations. His experience with pharmacology did not give him that feeling of that group. He wanted to be involved in helping the poor; all the goodness, all the good things that he would feel from a group; I don't think he got enough of that.

ESS: *Tell me, please, your understandings of what was troubling him. How do you account for the temper tantrums and the difficulties as a young child?*

DAD: My wife and I were married; we had our four children. His older brother was in therapy, as well. All the children were very bright children. The oldest tested genius, rating 200 in some areas, way off the board. Arthur was the little brother, he was very much left at the starting blocks as he was growing up. When the older brother was four, Arthur hardly spoke. When the older brother was six, Arthur hardly read. His older brother played basketball at ten years old, and Arthur hardly played anything.

ESS: *Was he ever called stupid or often compared directly with his older brother?*

DAD: Never. In my mind's eye I could only see it. Of course, it is obvious that the older brother was always praised and adored. This is hard not to do; he played in a Shakespeare play, and he knew all his lines, and all these things, when he was eleven. And he could read anything. He could write anything, and he could do anything, and, again, was physically attractive.

ESS: *So there was a real sibling difference?*

DAD: All I could see was that it was unfortunate for the little guy to have this big guy two years older having developed so quickly so well.

ESS: *Do you think that was one of the things that bugged him?*

DAD: And, in addition, his mother tends to be, at times, rather rigid. Her way of having the kids go to sleep at a certain time, eat at a certain time, eat a certain amount; all these things. I was raised in a very laissez-faire atmosphere at home. My whole stimulation for academic and personal excellence came from the peer groups.

ESS: *Do you think the imposition of that rigid program bothered Arthur?*

DAD: Of course it did. Only so much candy, only so much this, only so much that. He would become furious and enraged and fight

ESS: *It bugged him in a way that was different from the way it affected his older brother?*

DAD: His older brother would more or less go along with it or say some words. Arthur would go into a rage against her rules.

ESS: *What was the divorce about, and how public was it in the household, in front of the children?*

DAD: I would say they knew hardly anything about it. Right now I'm getting divorced from my second wife and seeing my first wife quite a lot.

ESS: *With the prospect of remarrying?*

DAD: A definite possibility.

ESS: *Brought together in part by Arthur's death?*

DAD: Definitely, yes, definitely. We have a lot in common. We were camp sweethearts.

ESS: *You have the most tragic thing in life in common.*

DAD: And I've known her for forty-five years. No surprises. Disappointments? I know she has a protective shield around her; her protective shield that she did nothing that was extraordinary for any parent, that would be damaging to Arthur. You asked me some questions about how people reacted. I'm saying that the regimen in the home was far too rigid. I come from a home where there wasn't that rigidity. Looking at it today, from what the professionals are saying, Arthur had a chemical imbalance that would make his response exaggerated to a normal stimulus. I don't know well enough, was it sixty/forty, seventy/thirty, eighty/twenty, ninety/ten, or reverse. I would say that sixty-five percent was home, thirty-five percent was his nature.

ESS: *In your own mind you perceive this as genetical, kind of an inborn predisposition, heightened reactivity?*

DAD: I do now, but I question a lot of that. I think the whole society is more receptive to using medicine to help balance people.

ESS: *You think that the therapist missed this?*

DAD: Seeing that Arthur tried to commit suicide when he was fourteen, and everything that was so much in place for Arthur from age fourteen until he finally killed himself, I think he definitely missed that. Because therapy was available for him, but there was something in his chemical makeup that took over. I personally feel that there are four parts to it. I feel there has to be the chemical part, just like any human being looking at an opera or going to the movies, whatever it is, there is something in your makeup that makes you excited, enthusiastic, or not. And so that part of his personality. The other thing would be the things he ate. I know he ate awful, I don't know if you have been told that. He was a meat and potatoes guy, no vegetables or fruits. There may have been something in that eating. He rejected food very early on and also emotionally; and he couldn't go out and have a pizza until he was sixteen or seventeen.

ESS: *Because?*

DAD: Because he wouldn't eat most of the things on a pizza. Finally, he could have a pizza. He didn't eat a salad in his whole life, never a salad. He didn't like it and of course became repulsed by it, but he lived with this all his life. He didn't like the taste. But I think, again I don't know, but I think part of this was to his mom's regimen. In my house, when I grew up, my mother just put it on the table, and we ate what we wanted. There was never a "you need to eat your vegetables, your protein, your dessert."

ESS: *Did you fight about these things?*

DAD: It's so many years ago. I'm sure that I was relatively passive those years. I just saw her as perfection. But when things were going wrong with the kids, like going to sleep at a certain time, and there was such a rebellion, to me, so what if he got to school in the morning and he didn't sleep through class, let him stay up.

ESS: *What finally happened?*

DAD: She wanted a divorce. But ultimately it wasn't changing, so I divorced her, but I was hoping that it would change.

ESS: *You had four things in mind.*

DAD: Yes, also physical exercise would be another thing. He became very physically active for a while, and I think that may have given him more balance. Another one was interactive therapy, talking to someone and just saying the words: I'm unhappy, I'm this, and getting somebody to talk to instead of keeping it all inside of him. Our home has always been both a philosophical, thoughtful home where we talked values; about the idea of death and so forth. I know that, in the last year or so before he killed himself, he was studying religion and the whole idea of the afterlife and the purpose of life, and he was discussing this with his older brother. They became very close friends in the last few years. As I said, his older brother is brilliant; Arthur obviously was brilliant. They could talk on a very high level. His older brother had no idea that inside Arthur he was looking at this from a different vantage point. It wasn't just for mental exercise. We always talked about this as a mental exercise, what is life's purpose, why give to charity, why go to the moon, just like normal people talk. But Arthur apparently was pursuing this because of his inner pain.

ESS: *Tell me what you think that pain was.*

DAD: I can only say from what he wrote in his last notes to us. He said there was a pain that was insufferable, it was almost constant, it was like knives being driven through his body.

ESS: *That describes the nature of the pain. What was the pain of?*

DAD: What was the cause? You mean, like pain of loneliness, pain of abandonment? I know that he did go into depths of depression again, afterwards, after he got divorced from his wife, probably also during high school or when he had such a wonderful weekend and then tried to commit suicide because he was going back to the lack of excitement of that wonderful weekend. After he divorced his wife, even though he was miserable in his life with her, I heard afterwards, he then went into deep depression. After he broke up with his girlfriend who, to me, was his real love, his soul mate; or, she may have broken up with him; he would always reject her at times. In his death note, he said, "I could go back to you, and maybe give me six months of joy but I know I would torture you again, and you mean too much to me." I don't think it was the pain of abandonment, of loneliness, of being inconsequential, or lack of achievement. It was the pain of constant depression. Pain no matter what he is doing, that he would have this demon inside of him that's tugging at him.

ESS: *Is it the pain of pessimism?*

DAD: No, pessimism is that I am going to fail with my family or my job.

ESS: *Is it the pain of dysphoria, the opposite of euphoria, that the world is dark?*

DAD: Well, I would say the lack of being able to have pleasure, because, even though he could be having a good time, he could only see it from the outside, that, "I'm smiling but I'm not really feeling good." And it was becoming more difficult for him, he said in his note, it was more difficult to function. I would think a fear of failure; that he was going to make a major mistake and be found out. It was also fear of the stigma that they'd find out that he was a crippled human being and they would reject him. If he could no longer be a doctor, then what would he do? Sell shoes? What could he do? He was at such a high level. They wouldn't permit him to continue if they knew that he was so troubled and it was so difficult making decisions. Ultimately, he'd make a wrong decision and someone would die, and he would be unmasked. I think that. Am I saying something that makes sense?

ESS: *You are saying something very powerful. I've not heard it verbalized so pointedly.*

DAD: It was in the note, but this is what I'm drawing from it, that he couldn't see himself being a fifty-, sixty-, or seventy-year-old person bearing this constant pain. You asked what the pain was, and I think that the pain would be that something would go drastically wrong and he would be found out. Because he kept it so secret. I would go to breakfast with him every Sunday morning. I would drive into the city to his apartment. He would call me, because if he wasn't available, I would call him the day before. He was a medical student, then an intern, then a law student; of course he was busy, he was overwhelmed, he was depressed, all within the normal sphere. So I couldn't see that it was exaggerated. When he called me we'd get together, and this was almost every Sunday. We'd just talk as father and son. We would talk about cases and colleagues. So, with me, we had wonderful Sundays, for an hour or so, until he said: "Well, got to go." And I'd say, "Have a good day, Arthur, you take care of yourself." He never shared with me what his pain was. About the note, we don't have just that last suicide note; we have his attempt about a year or two before. He wrote another six or eight pages, and that's where he mentions the camp experience and how he tried to kill himself because he had just had such a high time and he would have to go back into the pain. I was totally ignorant about the severity of this. All I could see was that he seemed happy until medical school, and then I assumed he was okay. His sisters and his mother knew enough, looking from now, but during that time his one sister knew that he had attempted suicide, and Arthur had sworn her to secrecy.

ESS: *Do you feel that it would have been draconian for his mother to take him out of medical school or law school and to put him in the hospital as a patient?*

DAD: I believe that. The only person it wouldn't be draconian for would be the psychiatrist and psychologist to have been attempting to do it the way his mother, who is also a therapist, would have involved herself in this wonderful young man's life. Arthur told his sister:

"I'm too smart to be kept in a hospital. I'll be out in a couple of days. I'll play the game, and I'll do what I choose to do anyway, so don't you dare try to hospitalize me." But again, if there is anyone who I am furious with, it was these highly trained, highly educated specialists; and Arthur wasn't a shoe salesman; he was a wonderful, special human being.

ESS: *What should they have done?*

DAD: They should have known that this was someone who could do harm to himself, and they could have called him.

ESS: *You are implying that his life should have been saved?*

DAD: No, I'm not. I'm saying that something could have been done that might have made a difference. I want to believe that his life could not have been saved; that's easier for me. I want to say that he was so deep into this that no one could have done anything; he would have found a way to have finished himself. But this doesn't give me any reason to not be angry and to not find incompetence. A therapist should keep the person alive, that's the main thing. And they failed. A string of them failed. Unbelievable. He got off his medications, you know that, like six months before he died; so between that time he was going through all kinds of emotional depression. Again, reconstructing: about three to four weeks before he died, he said to me: "Dad, I am really not happy with anything right now. I don't like school, I don't like the girls, nothing gives me any happiness." So I just said: "You know, Arthur, just take your time. There'll be a girl for you before you know it. You'll get into an easier situation, just, basically, suck it in and make believe in the meantime." And he also said, "When I'm with a girl on a date, and the girl says: 'Well, how is it being a doctor or a lawyer,' you want to say: 'Shit, I don't like it.' But you can't say that, so I fake it for a while; tell her I love being a doctor and a lawyer. Just a human talking." Looking back, I should have said to him, "Do you want to go to a hospital? Do you want to see a therapist?"

ESS: *Those were taboo, weren't they?*

DAD: I don't know. I could have said, "How can I help?" I don't know. But he would have said, "I can take care of myself."

CONSULTATION BY ROBERT E. LITMAN, M.D.

The story goes that Norman Farberow and I were having a recruitment cocktail hour with Dr. Litman at Trader Vic's in Los Angeles. Norm asked Bob if he would like another drink, and at that moment I asked Bob if he would join us as our chief psychiatrist at the Los Angeles Suicide Prevention Center, which we were in the process of forming. Bob said yes (to this date we're not sure whether it was to rum or suicidology). Dr. Litman, who was born 1921, is a product of Minnesota. His undergraduate degree and medical degree are both from the University of Minnesota. He also holds a Ph.D. from the Southern California Psychoanalytic Institute, and for years he has been the brilliant, effective, practical, productive, stimulating psychiatrist-in-chief at the LASPC. In his turn, he has been president of the American Association of Suicidology. In the recent past, he has had major heart surgery; he hardly had the energy to do this consultation, but he completed it as a labor of love to me and, more important, to his lifelong devotion to the pursuit of further knowledge relating to suicide. When I'm in trouble, I seek out his counsel.

In the 1960s, with our colleagues at the Los Angeles Suicide Prevention Center (SPC), we conceptualized suicide as a crisis, and our treatment model was crisis intervention. We thought of the presuicidal state as one of transient perturbation following trauma or serious loss, especially the loss or threat of loss of something that the patient valued highly. We emphasized the necessity for helping people get through these time-limited stress periods so that natural healing could occur. Much of our clinical work was based on the development of a 24-hour call-for-help crisis-intervention telephone service at the SPC, along with a program that provided a limited number of follow-up interviews for clients there, if needed. From the beginning, the telephone service was used extensively in Los Angeles, and the concept became so popular that crisis telephone services proliferated worldwide and spun off large numbers of hot lines for many purposes.

We wondered what happened to clients after they had been in touch with the emergency telephone service. Follow-up studies indicated a suicide mortality of about 1% after 2 years. Psychological autopsies revealed that, when these (now deceased) clients had called the SPC, they had been chronically psychiatrically ill and chronically suicidal. When asked what precipitating stress had caused them to call the SPC, these chronically suicidal clients often said, "Nothing special. I'm just tired of it all." They had difficulty recalling a specific time at which the suicidal state began. Although they had apparently called for help, they often were unwilling to accept the help that was suggested. Typically, these persons had a long history of chronic or repetitive suicidal behavior as part of a self-destructive lifestyle. They were chronically depressed. Some had made repeated suicide attempts. Many had disturbed personal relationships. Drug and alcohol abuse were common. Their suicidal behaviors did not represent crises as much as they represented repetitive behavior patterns. We learned that the treatment plan for these persons should emphasize the gradual amelioration of self-destructive lifestyles, with less emphasis on active intervention, to ensure their safety. The most effective intervention was to help these people find a stable and continuing treatment resource and encourage them to stick with it.

In the typology of suicide, Arthur represents a group of chronically suicidal persons who have talent and opportunity but are their own worst enemies. Arthur may well have called a crisis clinic and talked to a counselor, or his family may have called about him. Certainly, we encountered many such persons at the SPC. We had training tapes of interviews with them. A man demands, "Give me one reason that I should go on living." A woman says, "I know good things happen to me, but they don't stick to my stomach."

Persons who have had some experience with mental health treatment but who have dropped out of treatment make up about 25% of all the suicides, according to psychological autopsy research. Arthur has had a great deal of mental health treatment from one or more psychotherapists over a long period of time, as well as from a psychiatrist who prescribed medicine. Both the psychotherapy and the medicines were helpful. In trying to unravel the complex network of causation in this suicide, my experience leads me to focus on why Arthur rejected the treatment that had been helpful. In his note, he says that he rejected treatment because it provided only temporary relief and because he knew his pain would return; therefore, with apologies to the various people who helped him and loved him, he chose to avoid further pain by committing suicide.

Is mental pain (psychache) the central issue in this suicide, or is the major factor his inability or unwillingness to endure and overcome his pain? Shneidman has decided that psychache is the mother lode of suicidal thoughts and actions. Relieve the psychache and prevent the suicide. I have argued that, often, the psychological structure of help rejection is more important, or at least must be dealt with first for suicide prevention. Arthur was a physician. He knew that multimillions of people suffer from depression and get some help from treatment, but he felt that his pain was of a different order from that of other people, and his eventual fate was different from that of other people. He was uniquely doomed, in his mind. There was a profound narcissistic grandiosity in this way of thinking. When Arthur said to his estranged girlfriend that she must come back to him to love him or he would kill himself, he illustrated the mind-set of the multitalented suicidal person: "My way or no way."

In treating talented, chronically suicidal patients long term, I try to discover their guiding dreams and fantasies and hook their narcissistic attention to their own imaginative selves (the point is to make unconscious guiding fantasies conscious). Like Scheherazade with the fabled sultan, I try to fascinate them with the riddles of their dreams and imaginations so that they postpone the ending (suicide) in order to satisfy their curiosity about themselves. And as soon as I can, I try to persuade them to experiment with antidepressant medicine. Arthur seems to have had a guiding fantasy of rescuing and being rescued by a beautiful, perfect woman who would create sexual desire and satisfaction for him and make life worth living.

The interviewer, Dr. Shneidman, is tactful but curious, asking people about Arthur's sexuality. The wife says that they did not have intercourse before they got married and that, after they got married, it was not a big deal; it was very seldom. Arthur himself seems to have been disappointed that he wasn't sexually stimulated by his wife, and eventually they were divorced. The situation was repeated with a very attractive girlfriend whom he tried to seduce; then, even though they had a sexual relationship, he didn't seem to value it.

The interview with the psychotherapist doesn't tell us much about Arthur's sexual fantasies. Did he ever masturbate? When he entered medical school, what did it mean in his imagination? He wrote notes. He wanted to communicate. It is possible that an experienced and skilled suicidologist-therapist could have postponed Arthur's suicide, perhaps indefinitely. Maybe Ed Shneidman, in his prime, could have been successful in bringing about a five-year or a ten-year "cure." But there is a strict limit to how many of these suicidal patients any therapist can have in treatment at a time. It is important that the personal life of the therapist is in order, because this kind of treatment is a marathon, and it can be exhausting. If the exhaustion starts to show, the treatment ends.

At times I was a faculty psychiatrist asked to treat troubled medical students. I found that treating a suicidal medical student who carried the hopes and aspirations of family and school was stressful. For me, it was essential to use a team approach in the treatment of suicidal patients, and I would discuss cases with my colleagues rather continuously when there was a high suicide risk.

An important problem in suicide prevention is that there are many chronically suicidal persons in the world and limited resources to treat them with psychotherapy. That is why we turn so hopefully to psychopharmacology for help.

CONSULTATION BY
JEROME MOTTO, M.D.

Dr. Motto did his residency in psychiatry at Johns Hopkins in the '50s. For more than thirty years he ran a ward for suicidal patients at the University of California at San Francisco, where he was professor of psychiatry and is now, since 1991, professor emeritus. He has published 85 works on suicide and suicide prevention. He has been president of the American Association of Suicidology. He has been cited as one of the best doctors in the country, and, in my mind, he is one of the best suicidologists ever. He is a model of integrity and professional wisdom and has a reputation for writing the most thorough clinical reports in existence.

The Event

We are examining the suicide of Arthur, a 33-year-old Caucasian male physician and attorney. His death on a Sunday night resulted from an overdose of medication. On the day of his suicide, he spent time with his best friend and had a customary Sunday breakfast with his father. Neither of them detected anything unusual in his demeanor that might have presaged his impending action. He left a long and compassionate suicide note, apparently started on the preceding Friday night, that eloquently illustrates why he was characterized by some who knew him well as a loving and articulate man. In the note, he is very supportive of his surviving friends and family, imploring them: "Please, I beg you to celebrate for me that I can be free of pain."

The Background

Arthur's growth and development had been anything but normal. He was born into a middle-class family—his father was a physician, his mother a stay-at-home mom; he had two younger sisters and a brother 2 years older. Though his mother described him as "a very sweet little boy," by the age of 2 he was subject to "horrible temper tantrums." He would scream, yell, and be very difficult to manage. He didn't speak till he was nearly 3, and then he started speaking in sentences. In kindergarten, he had a "very sweet demeanor," but "could go very wild and crazy," once knocking his teacher's glasses off. Such episodes were triggered by the least provocation, and his mother realized over the years that he showed an extreme overreaction to anything that upset him in any way. His reading facility was delayed till age 7 or 8, and he sucked his thumb till age 9, requiring headgear for orthodontic treatment. That his behavior mirrored severe internal distress was made clear by his best friend, who recalled that at age 7 Arthur told him, "One day I'll kill myself." At the same time, he was seen to be creative, adept with his hands, and curious in exploring his environment. He appeared to be always in competition with his older brother, who was unusually gifted both physically and intellectually, and who, in the early years, would often bully Arthur, who thought his father favored the older son.

Arthur had very rigidly structured eating habits, described as meat and potatoes only, never eating a salad. He realized the strangeness of this and was embarrassed by it. At age 10, "he'd come crying to his mother, saying, Why can't I eat pizza like the other kids? What's wrong with me?"

Arthur's early school experience was so tumultuous that by the third grade, at age 8, he began psychotherapy twice weekly. The therapist describes him as "one of the angriest children I have ever seen"— "physically almost unmanageable"—"one of the most difficult children I have ever seen." Treatment apparently went well, however, and after Arthur improved "dramatically" and things were going well in school, treatment was terminated.

Arthur showed a long-standing animosity toward his mother, who divorced his father when Arthur was 10 years old. The divorce appeared to increase his hostility, yet he seemed to remain dependent on her and turned to her first when under stress. Arthur's therapist opines that something went awry very early in the bonding between the two of them and that the problem never went away. She saw Arthur's behavior toward her as his way of expressing all his frustrations, with daily violent tantrums that required her to restrain him physically. Later, when out on his own, Arthur seldom saw his mother, though he saw his father regularly. His father felt the mother was too rigid with all four children, and his mother felt she had devoted more than 30 years to trying to care for Arthur "as a special person who lived a very tormented life."

At the age of 12, after receiving an A+ on a school project, Arthur improved markedly in school and with friends and teachers. Thus it came as a surprise when, at the age of 15, after a very positive experience at a weekend camp, Arthur made a serious suicide attempt by overdosing on Tylenol. He later explained that the time at camp was so wonderful that he couldn't face returning to the "torture day after day in school," where he frequently thought of suicide. Though he saw no one as being cruel to him there, he felt very isolated and alone. After this episode, he returned to psychotherapy and seemed to improve again, graduating from high school with many friends and with academic honors.

Though his mother had been told informally that Arthur had a learning disability, it was not till college that this was identified as an "auditory discriminatory problem," such that he could not learn by auditory input but learned readily by reading. Despite this handicap, he went on to make Phi Beta Kappa and top honors in medical school and law school. Though acknowledging his successes, he tended to minimize them, downplaying his academic ability and even ascribing his admission to medical school to the fact that his then wife (already a medical student) talked to key persons on his behalf.

While in medical school, he called his therapist and initiated a third period of psychotherapy after a lapse of several years. He was seen to be quite depressed, with severe feelings of inadequacy as a student and as a potential physician. He also struggled with intense guilt related to being unhappy with his wife, whom he felt he had married hastily due to his own insecurity and need to be with somebody.

Though he was experiencing suicidal ideas during this period of treatment, Arthur worked through the separation from his wife and their divorce. He accepted antidepressant medication (which he felt helped him dramatically) from a psychiatrist, graduated from medical school and then law school, and began a new relationship with a girl-friend. When psychotherapy was again discontinued, he was described as functioning without difficulty and with improved self-confidence. In a follow-up telephone call, Arthur reported that he was feeling well and that things were going well, though his best friend observed that Arthur supplemented his medication with "some stuff from the hospital and he shot himself up with Demerol or something."

As might be anticipated, Arthur's relationship with his girlfriend followed a pattern similar to that with his wife: After an apparently happy year with her, he declared that he was no longer happy and broke off their relationship. However, he missed her so painfully that after 2 weeks he called her to ask if they could get back together, which she agreed to. There followed a series of repeated separations and reconciliations. Each breakup was initiated by Arthur and was subsequently resolved by his calling his girlfriend and pleading with her to take him back, only to reiterate his lack of happiness after a few months and break off their relationship again. The girlfriend clearly cared for him a great deal, but she was also pressured by Arthur's repeated statements that if she didn't take him back, he would kill himself. In time, the breakups became less traumatic for her, along with a growing conviction that whether or not they were together, Arthur would eventually commit suicide. She finally told him that she could no longer continue in this way, and they remained apart, though Arthur continued to call her.

Two or three weeks before his death, Arthur confided to his father that he was finding no joy in anything, a state of anhedonia that his father attributed to Arthur having gone off his medications some months earlier. He encouraged Arthur to persevere, assuring him that things would change for the better.

Late on the Friday night before his death, Arthur called his girl-friend to plead with her to take him back, again saying, "If you don't get back together with me, I'm going to kill myself." She took this threat seriously, as she had the many prior times she had heard it; after they had conversed for an hour, Arthur promised not to act on it. The next morning (Saturday), she called him "to make sure he was doing okay," and found him "like his normal self," in a good mood, and planning to go out with his best friend. The following day (Sunday), after seeing his best friend again and visiting with his father, Arthur ingested a lethal overdose, leaving the suicide note described.

The Problem

The problem at hand is an unusual one. It is not a question of cause of death, clearly an overdose; nor of mode of death, well documented by the deceased as a suicide; nor even of the motivation for the death, relief from unbearable pain, also well documented not only by Arthur in his suicide note but also by the remarkably consistent testimony of those who knew him well. The problem is rather how to understand the source of that motivation, the seemingly ever-present experience or anticipated recurrence of an excruciatingly painful emotional state—graphically described to his sister "as if someone was hammering nails into him every second into every part of his body" and to his girlfriend "like lying on a bed of needles." Such a complaint by a suffering person is so unusual that it presents a unique challenge to find a plausible explanation for it, a challenge made no easier by the fact that the experience apparently dated from very early childhood.

An Etiological Perspective

It seems clear that the painful existence from which Arthur finally freed himself had begun by the age of 2. Those who knew him well state confidently that "he was born with it." His therapist explained it as stemming from "a biological, physiological vulnerability," and his psychiatrist called it "a biological curse" that was not curable.

The diagnostic term that might best explain his behavior and experience is autistic disorder, first described by Kanner (1943) and characterized by a wide range of behavioral symptoms.[1] These symptoms tend to be associated with a common observation that, by the age of 3, the individual seems to be living in a private world, which markedly affects his or her interaction with the world outside. The *DSM-IV* (American Psychiatric Association, 1994) lists among the early signs delayed speech, aggressiveness, and—particularly in young children—temper

---

[1]On a personal historical note, I am reminded that Leo Kanner, who first described "early infantile autism" (also known as Kanner's syndrome) in 1943, was my supervisor in my residency in 1953 at Johns Hopkins University, during my child psychiatry rotation.

tantrums. An oversensitivity and exaggerated reaction to sensory stimuli—touch, sound, light, odors—is also described, as are abnormalities in eating, such as limiting diet to a few foods.

The hypersensitivity to stimuli has been focused on by clinicians to explain why autistic individuals may try to relate to the world about them but repeatedly withdraw from it again. This reaction is attributed to the world being too stimulating, and, because they are excruciatingly sensitive to stimuli, they are forced to retreat. This extreme sensitivity has been termed *sensory integration disorder*. One aspect of the sensitivity to touch has been expressed thus: "Imagine yourself in clothes so irritating that they seem lined with metal scraping brushes" (Stacey, 2003). One wonders if this sensitivity is related to some of Arthur's descriptions of his pain.

The *DSM-IV* (1994) anticipated another diagnostic issue pertinent to Arthur's experience in observing that, in adolescence or early adult life, individuals with autistic disorder who have the intellectual capacity for insight may become depressed in response to the realization of their serious impairment. Arthur may have been especially vulnerable in view of his mother's statement that she had a tendency to depression and that her mother did, as well. Arthur puts it in rational terms: "I am seeing that my problems were not as temporary as I imagined—they are quite permanent—I cannot hide from them or shake them—(the life that I envision) would not be a life worth living."

However labeled, it is clear that Arthur's lifelong pathology was paired with some remarkable strengths. His intelligence and insight were clearly demonstrated, and, in the course of his valiant struggle to overcome his disorder, he was described by others as tough, articulate, compassionate, funny, sweet, big-hearted, hardworking, loving, nurturing, a really good man, and a mensch. This may be considered ample evidence of a life well lived, however short and painful.

A Clinical Perspective

The two clinicians who treated Arthur saw him as a challenging patient with a guarded prognosis who apparently improved readily with treatment and was discharged with limited follow-up. His therapist saw him at crisis periods at ages 8, 15, and 28, and his psychiatrist saw him three times over a 5-month period at age 28. It appears that he was not in treatment for the 2½ years before his death, though some medications were apparently used. One could raise the question of whether a chronically suicidal individual should be monitored at regular intervals, even if stable, rather than waiting for another crisis. If medications helped as much as the record suggests, we must wonder why Arthur was not taking them during his last 6 months (according to his father).

A basic concept in treating suicidal persons is that a suicidal act can be expected if the person's level of psychic pain—or anticipated pain—exceeds the person's threshold of pain tolerance. Thus the pain level and pain tolerance thresholds require ongoing monitoring, as both are prone to fluctuation. In the situation at hand, Arthur's pain level could have been sharply increased by his girlfriend's refusal to accept him back on the Friday night on which he started writing his suicide note. At the same time, his threshold of pain tolerance may have been reduced by an invisible but often critical precipitant of suicide in high-functioning persons—emotional fatigue. If not relieved, a stress that was long coped with in the past can generate increasing fatigue, which gradually reduces the pain tolerance level till it is exceeded by the pain level; thus a suicide occurs with no visible warning. In this instance, Arthur's sounding and appearing "his usual self" to his ex-girlfriend and to his father and best friend on the day of his suicide would thus be understandable. As his sister summed it up, "He just couldn't take it any more."

The girlfriend's role is reminiscent of Shneidman's emphasis on the crucial role of the significant other in suicidal adults. As Arthur expresses it in his suicide note, "Right now I am sinking—drowning—she is all I feel can save me."

Another element in Arthur's situation is the possibility that his autistic disorder prevented the introjection of meaningful relationships that provide an essential stabilizing influence on emotional life. Referred to as a "sense of connectedness" or a "delusion of fusion," this critical element is not realized on a conscious level. Thus, for Arthur, gratifying relationships tended to be a transient experience; this fact may help account for his distant relationship with his mother and even his existential nihilism, expressed as, "Life just doesn't mean much to me, it's boring, I don't see the point, why bother?"

The clinical challenges presented by Arthur's lifelong disorder and its effect on his thinking, feelings, and behavior would be daunting even to the most experienced clinician. Those who saw him certainly helped him through some difficult crises. Regretfully, they were not called on when the final crisis developed.

Discussion and Conclusions

The chronic etiological issues here suggest an autistic disorder with an associated severe hypersensitivity and inability to internalize relationships, combined with intermittent depressive episodes that are excruciatingly painful, complicated by progressive emotional fatigue that diminishes the will and energy needed to continue, in an individual who has embraced the prospect of suicide since childhood. If we accept these issues, then what might have been done to make Arthur's life more bearable?

One consideration might have been to have remained in touch with Arthur for an indefinite period. Assuming he were doing well and no longer a candidate for psychotherapy, this could have taken the form of a brief telephone call every couple of weeks, initiated by the clinician, and informally structured to answer the question, Do things continue to go well?

If Arthur had responded to antidepressant medication, the dose might have been gradually tapered to a maintenance level and continued as in other chronic conditions, such as epilepsy or diabetes. If such medications ceased to be effective, a mood-elevating agent such as dextroamphetamine sulfate could have been considered, limiting the dose to a maximum of 30 milligrams per day. If no medication seemed to help but Arthur had gotten relief from a drug such as Demerol (which he was apparently taking on his own), this would have deserved consideration, with careful documentation and consultation to address any ethical issues. If no pharmacological agents could control handicapping symptoms, electroconvulsive therapy could be tried, with the possibility of a monthly maintenance schedule.

With Arthur's consent, it would have been desirable to meet with his family, to respond to their questions, to provide support, and to prepare them for the unpredictable outcome in such cases. Granted, the chances of Arthur having accepted these considerations do not appear to be very good.

Finally, there is no way to know whether Arthur's suicide might have been preventable. It might well have been delayed, as the psychiatrist interviewee suggested. The prominent biological basis of autism limits the effectiveness of psychological measures, and there are no medications specific to this disorder.

The most realistic response to the question about whether more could have been done is probably that voiced by one of Arthur's sisters. She reminds us that, for a 7-year-old who talks about killing himself to live to the age of 33, a great deal of help must have been given to him; that without the help of his family, loving others, and a therapist and without medication, he would have killed himself much earlier, but that "all the things we did do prolonged his life." She unknowingly speaks to many instances in which a suicide is seen as a failure, when in fact the length of life attained could be considered a triumph for the caregivers. Arthur's life—and death—deserve to be included among these.

CONSULTATION BY NORMAN L. FARBEROW, PH.D.

*During that marvelous, exciting period, in the 1950s and '60s, when we practically invented and certainly developed suicidology, Norman Farberow and I worked assiduously together as buddies and colleagues. Along with Dr. Robert Litman, we founded, directed, and ran the Los Angeles Suicide Prevention Center; we edited two pioneer books—*Clues to Suicide *(1957) and* The Cry for Help *(1961)—and several chapters and papers. Farberow was born in 1918, was an undergraduate at the University of Pittsburgh, and earned his Ph.D. from UCLA. He has been president of the American Association of Suicidology and has won awards and honors from local and international suicide organizations. He has spent most of his professional life as a director of the Los Angeles Suicide Prevention Center. He is currently professor emeritus (clinical) at the University of Southern California School of Medicine. He is certainly one of a half dozen premier suicidologists in the country, and I count him as one of my most important lifelong professional colleagues.*

Why Did Arthur Kill Himself?

Arthur's suicide was the result of a confluence of psychological factors with neurobiological and physiological factors. The most prominent of the psychological factors was a self-image in which he saw himself as inadequate, incapable, weak, and inferior. Those feelings about himself developed and were consistently reinforced during his childhood and adolescence. This self-concept of being worthless and undeserving of any love was primarily the result of the sibling rivalry that he developed with his brother, who was 2 years older and who he felt was preferred and favored by his parents. In his early childhood, his brother set an unattainable example of being bigger, smarter, brighter, speaking earlier, and walking earlier. In school, his big brother's example was one of brightness, intellectual abilities, academic achievements, good looks, social responsiveness, and athletic promise. Arthur showed none of these. He grew up with a feeling of being inferior in practically every sphere of his functioning. His response to the overwhelming sense of inferiority to his older brother was to engage in every way possible to garner attention, most of it negative. Preschool years were filled with violent, chaotic tantrums marked by rebellion against every effort to control him while he fought for evidence of love and acceptance. He was a miniature tornado who required close and constant watch to see that he did not hurt himself or others during his screaming tantrums. In school, he required consultations with his teachers, special arrangements for his attendance, and special home studies.

In addition, Arthur had a neuropsychological defect, an auditory learning disability that prevented him from discriminating sounds easily and understanding speech. He had difficulty learning anything that was presented orally, which probably contributed to his inability to speak until he was 3 years old. He was a poor physical specimen in his early years, small, scrawny, no match for his older brother, who physically bullied and overpowered him. He wore headgear to protect him from hurting his head during his tantrums, he had protruding teeth from sucking his thumb, and he wore glasses. The contrast in the amount of time and care required by each son must have been marked in the early years, with brother easy and compliant, whereas Arthur required constant vigilance and anxious worry.

As Arthur grew into adolescence and young adulthood, he became more fearful of his successes than he was of his failures. His successes were chimerical, undependable, and not to be believed. He coped with his successes by downgrading them or rationalizing that they were only temporary, so that any good feeling would shortly be overtaken by his reality of inescapable failure. He became skilled at procrastination, by which he could flirt with failure, which would only confirm his feelings; or he would succeed but at a lesser level than he was really capable of, allowing him to denigrate the success. The successes he had—and he had many, for he was bright—were only fragile masks behind which he felt it was impossible to hide. His constant fear was that he would make some horrible mistake and so would stand revealed for the inadequate, inferior person he really was. He felt that his entry into medical school was false and that he had cheated his way in by having his wife talk to the dean. Despite this feeling of failure, he was at or near the top of his class. Throughout his medical school years, he was afraid he would be found out, afraid of making some horrendous mistake, and that he would not be allowed to continue.

Why the suicide, and why now? Why did Arthur decide to end his life at this particular point? As his brother remarks, he seemed to be at a point in his life at which things were going well. He had been successful in his medical school studies; he was in his residency; he had a woman who understood him and was very much in love with him; and he had a family who, despite the many problems he had presented and the parents' divorce when he was about 10 years old, had been supportive and dependable during his troubled years. There was no indication of a "smoking gun," no specific event that shattered his world, no unexpected lethal blow to his fragile structure. His only concern was his chronic, unrelenting pain, heavy, pervasive, and unshakable.

He started writing his note on Friday. I suspect that he had spent most of Saturday writing his good-byes to his pal, his sister, and his girlfriend. It was not the first time he had been in this kind of position, in which he had decided to end his life, had begun to write his notes of explanation, and then had interrupted them. He makes references to how often in the past he had written similar notes, sometimes even making an attempt to escape the life he had found not worth living, only to continue on. This time he made the attempt with oxycontin, "finished" his note at 11:30 p.m., when he became drowsy, but unhappily woke up the next morning, not having taken enough to complete his effort. He vomited lithium, but it is unclear when he took the lithium, whether it was with the oxycontin or when he awakened that morning. He writes rationally about his earlier suicide attempt at 14 years of age, after his exhilarating "normal" experience in camp, one that he could not derive any integrated pleasure from. His return from camp only meant a return to the increasingly deeper unhappiness and pain that had been growing steadily unbearable.

Arthur had made a number of suicide attempts in the past, some of them quite serious, with the degree of ambivalence in them varying considerably. More recently, it seems that the level of his ambivalence had dropped and his attempts had become more lethal. At least one was close to fatal; he told the physician who monitored his case while he was in med school of his efforts to die the previous night by means of a plastic bag over his head. Although some ambivalence remained in his thinking on the fateful weekend, it was weak, and he had firmed his decision to die. His intentions remained strong, even though a number of events occurred that weekend that might well have helped him to survive. He had spent Sunday morning with his best friend, who had been privy to many of his severe bouts of depression in the past and who had helped him through them. This time Arthur gave him no indication of his most recent self-destructive actions or of his intentions to end his life that same night. Arthur was also in touch with his father at some time in that weekend and borrowed money from him, which, being scrupulously honest, according to his sister, he fully intended to repay. And he had been in touch with his ex-girlfriend, whom he had called Friday night to tell her he was going to kill himself. Because she had heard this threat many times before, she took no action in response. She was about to leave town, and he lied to her that he was not going to commit suicide. She called him on Sunday from the airport, and he even promised her he would not.

The ambivalence had been a critical factor throughout his relationship with her. He had looked to her to save him from himself. She had almost succeeded, for he had found her to be loving and caring and to give him great pleasure; but she was not able to win out over the depression that he lived with constantly. He looked to her to "force" him into environments that should have led him to contentment, but it would only mean another cycle of "honeymoon" period followed by torture. His ambivalence emerged in his statement that he could call his girlfriend and she would save him, but again, he would experience only temporary relief from his pain. The temptation was there to survive again as he thought about his girlfriend, but again the anticipation of the pain that was sure to follow made him hide his decision from her.

Family's Role in Arthur's Suicide

His mother was Arthur's primary source of care, but, in his early years, he was hardly a source of pleasure or joy for her. Arthur was in a constant state of rebellion marked by tantrums and destructiveness.

She had to use physical restraint when she could not calm him with words. Her efforts at some kind of control were expressed through restrictive rules and setting limits. She set schedules for the children for eating and for bedtime. There was great emphasis in the home on academics, and although she didn't push him, the expectation was there. Compared with his brother, Arthur learned that he was not good enough to be loved, that he was at most tolerated rather than loved, and he carried that sense of being a failure throughout his life. His mother's understanding of Arthur's condition was that it was mostly due to frustration. As a result, he was always angry, and he took out all his anger on her. He was frustrated by his brother, who overpowered him physically and took advantage of him in play. He was frustrated in school because he couldn't learn and because he could not live up to what was expected of him. His mother feels that Arthur blamed her for the divorce, but that the divorce didn't cause his problems, only exacerbated them. Being a mother to this "special person" who lived a tormented life was costly. In her own words, taking care of Arthur made a mess out of her life. It took up all her life for 30 years; she felt she could do nothing else but take care of her children. She feels she was cheated out of her right to get and to give love.

His father was not so crucial in Arthur's development. He feels neither blame nor guilt for Arthur's suicide. Arthur's fights were with his mother and his brother, not with him. He blames the mother's restrictive rules and the competition with his brother as contributing to Arthur's depression, but he himself also contributed to its development by his appreciation of the older brother's abilities, physical superiority, and athleticism. He recognizes Arthur's predicament but says that it simply was unfortunate for "this little guy to have this big guy 2 years older having developed so quickly so well." He attempted to fill the role of father. Even while separated, he would take custody of Arthur on alternate weeks, helping him when he could and participating with him in extracurricular games. Even so, he ended up primarily as a source of financial help and received little respect from Arthur.

His father's understanding of Arthur's suicide is mixed. He is somewhat simplistic in attributing the suicide to four basic factors: chemical, or something inherent; diet, because Arthur ate a limited variety of foods; physical, because Arthur was weak and scrawny as a child; and treatment, because his therapists did not do enough to keep him alive. On the other hand, he was aware of the degree to which Arthur felt he was a failure and suffered the constant fear of being exposed as a sham. He reverses the process by which the suicide occurred by attributing the feelings of loneliness, inconsequentiality, pessimism, and fear of failure to Arthur's depression instead of recognizing that it was those feelings that were the basis of his depression.

The older brother's interview provided more information about the family's functioning. He remembered Arthur as being afraid to try new things to eat for fear they would not be pleasant. He attributed Arthur's early activity, such as running away from home innumerable times and fighting against what he couldn't avoid, as defensive, as a way of avoiding things that might be painful. He was aware that competition with him was a vital part of Arthur's life. He simply took advantage of his extra 2 years, high intelligence, and physical ability to bully Arthur as they grew up. He asserted that he never felt competitive but admitted that Arthur worked so hard to improve himself that by the time he was in college he was able to surpass his brother in just about every way, whether it was in intellect, accomplishments, or social skills. Arthur's family was important to him. His brother feels that their parent's divorce, when Arthur was about 10, was a severe blow to him and made him feel that he did not have a normal family. The brother believes that it assaulted his sense of basic trust, giving him the feeling that his world was not trustworthy. His brother was hardly surprised over Arthur's suicide, just that it occurred when it finally did, when there were so many positive factors in his life, such as a loving girlfriend and success in his work. However, Arthur had two sides that he lived with, a dark side and a bright side. The dark side, the biological depression, finally won out.

The Compartmentalization of Success

Why didn't Arthur learn from his successes? Why was he not able to learn and to profit from his experiences of success? Was the suicide the result of a neurological or physiological disability that led him to believe that he was weak, underdeveloped, and uncoordinated, or was it the result of his conviction that he was an unredeemable failure? By the time Arthur was in his 20s, he had learned that he could succeed in almost anything he undertook, even though it might require huge effort. But none of his successes dispelled his core feeling of failure. That feeling might lie quiescent for a time, but it was always there and would always reappear, even while his successes continued. Arthur had begun to feel that the only way to overcome or to escape such failure was to kill himself. Members of his family may never have expressed it, but they also had come to believe that Arthur was doomed and that his suicide was inevitable. His father, sister, and brother believe it was "chemical"; his girlfriend and physician believe it was a "psychiatric malignancy." His psychotherapist feels that a biological explanation was most important and that biological factors were exacerbated by the difficulties he experienced in life. His best friend is the only one who believes that perhaps more positive experiences, maybe another positive relationship or possibly more medication, might help. There is no doubt that medication did help in relieving Arthur of some of his pain. But he always felt it would not last.

In my view, the therapist comes closest to the truth but has the emphasis wrong. I think that, to Arthur, the psychological aspect of his life was basic to his view of his life, and this belief was added to any neurological predisposition or deficiency. To function adequately in our culture requires that one has to learn to like, or at least to tolerate, oneself, warts and all. This is a learned process. One is not born with a poor self-image; one is taught that, in the same way that a good self-image is taught. The capacity for self-love, adequate self-image, and self-confidence is imparted to the individual by the major figures in his rearing, starting from day one. One may be born with neurobiophysiological defects, whether bodily, neurological, or chemical, but, assuming there is adequate intellect, they can be overcome, so that suicide is not the only and inevitable resolution. Arthur had the necessary intellect to learn. He may have had his share of a variety of deficiencies when he was born, but they need not have condemned him to such a miserable life. Arthur proved this by overcoming and correcting most of his physical difficulties. With his intellect, he was able to achieve the academic recognition he wanted, and hard effort and medicine overcame his physical problems of poor vision, denture distortions, and apparent lack of athletic ability. Arthur's early psychological experience of being "not as good as" branded him with a self-concept of inadequacy and failure. This became his "malignancy," which, along with his physical problems, became his reality. He saw this in every experience, so that it became an inevitability.

Why could it not be treated? It was. Medications helped in terms of their effect on his neurological functioning, lessening his weakened self-image. His early psychotherapy, starting when he was about 7 years old, supported the beginnings of a sense of self-value and independence, but these senses were rudimentary to begin with and could not overcome an already formed conviction of inadequacy. What Arthur lacked was trust, a faith that his world was secure, a belief that good feelings about himself were deserved and could last and overcome the image of worthlessness that had become his essence and that stalked every pleasure he was enjoying. How does this feeling of self-worth develop? It comes from the major figures in his world loving him and valuing him, despite any defects he may have been born with. It comes from feeling safe and protected, from having a haven to which he can always retreat and from which he can venture again to learn once more about his world. It does not come from a sense of obligatory, resentful caring or from devalued regard.

Could Arthur Have Been Saved?

Each interviewee was asked whether Arthur could have been saved. I believe he could have been. It would have required a therapist who firmly believed that he was worth saving, that the restructuring of Arthur's self-image was possible, and that Arthur was worth the investment of the effort, the time, and the energy. It would have required convincing Arthur that this was possible. It would have required that Arthur trust the therapist and his or her belief to the point of being willing to invest himself in the therapist's care and guidance. Medication would play a significant role, for the therapist would use it for both medical and psychological support.

There is some evidence that this kind of approach had already succeeded in the past. Arthur had made a number of suicide attempts in the past, most of them bound by ambivalence, some of them bound by fear that he would end up even more damaged than he was. Medication alone would not have sufficed, for it would not have changed the basic feelings he had about himself, nor would it have affected his concept of himself as a failure. What was needed was the combination of perceptive, patient, and persevering psychotherapy with the mutually determined objective of change in self-concept, along with medication to help him over the inevitable rough spots.

INTERVIEW WITH
THE BROTHER

ESS: *Here we go. How much older than Arthur are you?*

BRO: I was born 24 months before Arthur.

ESS: *Please tell me about him.*

BRO: [Sigh] It's hard to know where to begin. I was a couple of years older than Arthur, and we were a close family growing up, but Arthur and I fought a lot. I am somewhat ashamed and regretful of the fact that I bullied him a bit growing up, and I was regretful about that before he died. He and I. . . . I guess I'll skip over stuff and go back.

ESS: *Please.*

BRO: You know, he and I became closer as the years progressed; by the time he was twenty, he and I had become quite close, and, in fact, the year before his death, he and I lived together in an apartment here; and, I've verbalized this thought and I'll say it now, I considered him one of my best friends in the world, as well as my brother. He was a complex person, like everyone is.

ESS: *Apparently more than most.*

BRO: Probably so. He had a very difficult time as a child. Among other things, he wouldn't eat anything. He had serious issues with food. He was afraid to try new foods.

ESS: *Phobic?*

BRO: Maybe so. I mean, he was petrified about eating. He would only eat meat with no sauce on it, he wouldn't eat any vegetables, he wouldn't eat any fruits. My parents bribed him to eat. They would give him ten dollars to try lettuce.

ESS: *You use a strong word, petrified. Do you mean that?*

BRO: He was.

ESS: *What was he afraid of?*

BRO: That's hard to say. He was afraid, I can't say, he was afraid to try new foods, and I know it stigmatized him to some degree. He was afraid to go to friends' homes, in the fear that he would be embarrassed at having to turn down all the food offered at dinner. I don't think he was afraid he'd be poisoned. I think he was just afraid of the taste disagreeing with him so much. I don't think he had a paranoia about that.

ESS: *Was he afraid of being seen as flexible? Was he afraid to give up a position of, "This is the way I want things and no other way?"*

BRO: I don't know about that, because I think he was almost embarrassed about it. I remember that he would come to my mother, crying, when he was maybe eight or ten years old, saying, "Why can't I, why am I not like the other kids, why can't I eat pizza? What's wrong with me?" And, I mean it was a big breakthrough when he was maybe thirteen or fourteen and he finally, for a 20 dollar bribe from my parents, started eating pizza. But he was a very scrawny kid, and he also sucked his thumb till he was about 6 years old, when his teeth were pushed far out from it; he wore headgear, and he also was nearsighted, so he wore glasses when he was six, and he was awkward socially. He acted out in school. I don't think he was particularly violent, but he would just disrupt his classes, and he would try and run away both from school and from our home on numerous occasions

ESS: *How would he disrupt classes?*

BRO: I think he would make wisecracks off the things the teachers were saying.

ESS: *Would he shout obscenities?*

BRO: I don't know the answer to that. He wasn't a total pariah or anything like that. He had, there was some affection that was felt for him, I think, by both his classmates and his teachers, even though he was such a nuisance, and, finally, by the time he was 13 or 14 he started—I mean I was going to say he was becoming more comfortable with himself, but I don't know if that was it or not—but he developed friendships and a peer group at that time. He started working out; he got rid of his glasses—it was a big thing to wear contact lenses for the first time. He started becoming muscular and kind of played football. He, I mean this is hard for me to say and talk about but I know that, I know he felt he was in my shadow in a lot of ways, and I can say, you know, the odd thing is that in the couple of years before his death, I felt that he had surpassed me after starting so far behind in so many ways. I mean, I was a good athlete, and I was good in school and popular socially, and he was awkward in all these ways. And he also was more conservative than me, both in style and in politics—although he wasn't conservative politically—but, and it was always odd to people in our peer group that we had become so close in our twenties, because people would always say we seemed so different.

ESS: *Was he seen as a problem child?*

BRO: Yeah, he was seen as a problem child.

ESS: *Sort of a nerd?*

BRO: Not really; I mean, in a way yes until he was maybe twelve or thirteen and then no; he became quite popular. He was a good-looking kid. I mean he really had an awkward face up until the age of maybe twelve or so.

ESS: *Was he sort of your nerdy little brother who was a pain in the ass?*

BRO: Yeah, to some degree, and I, well, I enjoyed the power that I had over him, and—but then we became close, in our twenties, we became very close and, and, most of the things I'm going to say to you now I've said to my other good friends and family, just in talking about this over the years, but I mean, I felt like Arthur was the person that I felt most comfortable with in the world, and I felt he was the person whose mind worked most similarly to mine, and we talked about everything. Our main recreation was playing Scrabble; you know, we played Scrabble together nonstop by the hour. In his suicide note, he says, look through my stuff, which we did, and we found many other writings and notes that he had done over the years when he was feeling similarly. And it became clear that he had made several other suicide attempts that might have been half-hearted to some degree, that's hard to know, where he put a plastic bag over his head many times, trying to kill himself that way before going to sleep, and it not working, but then filing a lot of these notes away. And I have those notes, and then, and I was just mentioning, just in one of them he just spoke to me about regretting that we won't be able to grow old together over a Scrabble table.

ESS: *Do you have any thoughts about where he got that negative outlook on life, that happiness was not for him?*

BRO: When you say that happiness was not for him, that's apparent; objectively, that has to be accepted. I'm saying that the fact that he killed himself and—well, of course his death is enigmatic, but in looking at his note it's clear that on one level or another he felt that he was doomed to never be happy and that this was his only way out, that happiness was not for him, and he did feel that, clearly. What I am saying is that at the same time, he embraced life in many ways. It seems like he lived in parallel existences; one, just like planning on taking his own life at some point; one just like, whatever, I can do whatever I want to, because I'm going to end up killing myself, nothing matters; and another one, and they might have been related, where he embraced things; for example, one of the things that I found among his papers was "Tips to a Traveler," and he had written a list. Our families traveled a lot, and he and I did some traveling together in Europe, and he had made a list on traveling; and they were just suggestions that really showed an embracing of life and seeking experience. Examples: You don't want to stay in the finest hotels, you want to stay in a place where you can interact with some of the local people, and try to take public transportation when you can.

ESS: *So there was a "life" side to him.*

BRO: Oh yeah, and he was humorous, he was like a glib funny guy, you know, warm, in a warm kind of way; he was a warm, funny person.

ESS: *Did you find the presence of this dark side in him paradoxical and puzzling?*

BRO: Not really, just, sometimes at its furthest reaches I would. One of the main things you asked, where he might have gotten this dark and negative attitude, his pessimistic attitude, I can't say, but, you know, my parents' divorce, that was certainly a significant event, and that happened when I was twelve and he was ten.

ESS: *What do you think that did to him? What lessons, good and bad, did he learn from that?*

BRO: It affected us so differently, and I didn't have a sense of the way in which it affected him until our twenties when, in talking about it, he, at one point, said "God, Mom really fucked up, she divorced dad and now she is alone." I never thought about it that way; I never thought that my parents' divorce was a bad thing. I always felt that, my perspective was, my parents were different people, and they married when they were young, and it made sense that they were no longer together, and I felt fine about it. I had two houses to go to, I had two rooms, and I felt okay. If I was in denial about it, I don't know, I felt all right; but Arthur felt like he had lost, you know, that in his mind we didn't have a normal family. So he married, and it was easy analysis to say okay, now he is, at the earliest opportunity, trying to set things right by creating his own family.

ESS: *Do you think that that divorce was an assault on his notion of basic trust, that his world was no longer trustworthy?*

BRO: Yeah, I mean, that would make sense.

ESS: *Do you remember, was there a time before he was dour and pessimistic? How early do those [feelings] come in?*

BRO: Well, you, I imagine, heard about his overdosing when he was fifteen years old. I mean, that's very hard to say. It seems, and again, some of these things are secondhand, but just a few weeks ago, I heard an anecdote about a teacher of his, when he was maybe 12, how Arthur, at that age, had made some joke or reference to strangling himself in the blinds at school. And then, his closest friend, as he was growing up, after Arthur died, talked about how Arthur had said that he would kill himself some day, since the time when they were little kids. So, clearly, it was there in some way earlier.

ESS: *What was that episode or event of his attempting suicide at eleven or twelve or so, what was that about?*

BRO: Well, what I can say is this, first of all, at the time that it happened, he was fifteen, I was seventeen. I was told that he had contracted food poisoning and he would be back in a couple of days. As I look back, I can't remember my interaction with him after he came back from the hospital after a couple of days, but I know it was only a few years after that, that I was at my father's office and (it may have been only a couple of years after that) and I happened to open up a confidential letter that was addressed to my father. I don't know what prompted me to do it, but it made a reference to Arthur's suicide attempt; and I asked my parents about it.

ESS: *Did you then treat him any differently?*

BRO: Yeah, at that point I already had stopped bullying him; I had already stopped that, and I, and in the time after that suicide attempt which—I mean I guess nobody has told you the story, but I could tell you the story even if it is secondhand. I mean he apparently—he was in tenth grade in high school, and he had gone on a weekend retreat, I think, a social retreat of some sort, and he had come back from the retreat, and during the retreat he had a good time socially, as he put it, like he was having a really good time, and the prospect of returning to high school the next day, where he felt like a total outcast, where at every lunch break he would sit alone and he would pretend to read because he had no one to interact with—the prospect of returning to that after he had felt so good was so daunting that he took a bottle of pills. So he took the pills and then, as he later put it, he chickened out, and he called his therapist. He had a psychotherapist from the time he was eight years old. So apparently he called his therapist, who then called my mom, and, as Arthur later put it, it wasn't that he decided, "I don't want to die," he was just afraid of what would happen and chickened out because he could have crippled himself. As I've said, he and I became very close friends in the last eight or nine years of his life; I mean, very close, and he was very similar to me, liked to talk about philosophical theoretical prospects, and it's weird, it's hard to look back at it like this, but, among conversations over the years, he would say, "life is overrated, what's the point, why bother?" He would say stuff like that to me, and I would take it as a philosophical question, and my basic response was, "yeah, there is no reason to live other than the reasons you yourself come up with," and we would take it from there. I really thought that he was better. He seemed so confident and successful; he excelled professionally, he was a doctor and a lawyer.

ESS: *You discussed philosophic nihilism as an abstract topic.*

BRO: Yes.

ESS: *How much of a surprise was his death for you?*

BRO: It wasn't a total surprise. If I had gotten a call from Arthur saying that my sister had killed herself, that would have been a total surprise; but hearing that Arthur had done it, one of my initial reactions was, "he really did it." Like he wasn't just talking; he really meant it.

ESS: *In your own mind, how do you see Arthur's death? Do you see it as biological, genetical, psychological; how do you conceptualize it?*

BRO: Obviously, I'm totally speculating, but it seems that it may have been quite biological. One doctor who saw him at the hospital said Arthur's suicide was the worst case of pure depression that he had seen. Arthur was the worst case of depression that he had seen in his time. Arthur was very responsible; actually, he killed himself on a Sunday night; he went to work on Friday and killed himself on Sunday night, and that rings consistent with some of these thoughts I had.

ESS: *An implied question is: Do you think something might have been done? The question is: Could he have been saved?*

BRO: I tend to think, I mean, unfortunately, I guess, I somehow think yes.

ESS: *Who could have done what?*

BRO: Somehow, I could have stayed in close proximity to him. Actually, I moved away. I moved across the country three months before he killed himself. I didn't have any alarm. I saw Arthur a couple of weeks before he did it; but I also saw him over New Year's. He came to a party at the home of a friend of mine, and I remember this friend saying, "My God, Arthur has it all together"; he came there with an attractive woman that he was dating and was fit and strong and was having a good time. I did not see him deteriorate. And I also had my own issues, my own concerns. I was in somewhat of a funk myself. I definitely had my own experiences of depression; clearly, it was put into much clearer focus after Arthur died. I'm still there. My life has been on the surface—Arthur's dead now—but I can say that when he was alive, that our lives were going in completely different directions. We made totally different choices. I remember Arthur in college. Quite different. Just so different. I was a very fast learner, and I scored exceptionally well on the SAT, National Merit Scholar, and all this, and Arthur—I knew how to read when I was three and a half, with my grandmother. Arthur couldn't read till he was about 8 years old, just plodding along, you know, physically somewhat weak, socially uncomfortable. He got a girlfriend, finally, I guess the last year of high school or right as he was going into college. Arthur just studied and studied and studied; and he graduated Phi Beta Kappa. He would study every day; he had a tremendous work ethic.

ESS: *Sounds like the hare and the tortoise. Much more complicated.*

BRO: Of course. Yes, and that's the thing. First of all, I must say that I never felt competitive with him. I know he felt competitive with me. I guess, especially growing up, there was no competition, I was so far ahead. By the time before he died, I definitely had the thought at times that I am a bit of a failure and Arthur had been such a success. But I felt less badly about myself and more proud of him, like he had really succeeded. I felt okay with my choices, that I hadn't chosen to live a conventional life.

INTERVIEW WITH
THE SISTER

ESS: *With your permission, I'd like to ask you a couple of general questions and some specific ones. The general question is: What do you think went on? Why do you think your brother took his life? What can you tell us about him?*

SIS: I'm a sister of Arthur's.[1] Arthur committed suicide, that you know, and when you say why, what went on—he suffered his whole life. He was always in pain, and as much as we all felt we understood it, none of us really could understand it, because none of us was suicidal; and he was constantly in pain and constantly looking for something that would make him feel happier, would make him feel better. He tried all different kind of things. He went first to medical school, and then changed his mind, that didn't make him happy, so then he went to law school because medical school didn't make him happy, thinking that maybe law school might make him happy. He was single and dating and then got married and wasn't happy, so he got divorced. His whole life he was striving to find what would make him feel better and not feel the pain, and I think after trying all the things that he always thought—if I married, if I had a good career, if I have friends, if I have all these things—and once he obtained all these things, he realized that these things still weren't making him feel out of pain, then I think his hopelessness just completely consumed him, and he couldn't take the pain any more. In his letters he indicates he felt someone was hammering nails in every inch of his

---

[1]There is another sister, 2 years younger, who was abroad and unavailable to be interviewed.

body every second of the day. Nobody should have to take that, and he couldn't take it anymore. I don't think he wanted to die, but I think he just didn't want to have that pain, and there was no way he felt, being alive, that he couldn't have that pain, and to him killing himself was the only way not to have the pain that he had had for so many years.

ESS: *You said he had been like this ever since he was a child? How do you in your own mind account for this streak in him?*

SIS: I think it's just chemicals, not situational, something the way he was born, inside of him, you know, chemical makeup. We learned after he died that he knew his whole life. A best friend remembered when Arthur was seven, he said, "One day I'll kill myself," and that's not something that a 7-year-old says, it's not something that children that age even think about.

ESS: *Are there any other suicidal deaths in your family?*

SIS: No, nothing to my knowledge, no. If there is, then it's something in the very distant past, no family members I know about.

ESS: *I want to use the word* dysphoric, *negative, lugubrious, nay-saying, pessimistic. How early did you see this in your brother?*

SIS: You know what, we really didn't have a clue. You know, people get upset, people get depressed. People have problems, people get depressed, people get sad, people get tired, things like that, and I didn't know anything. Arthur tried to commit suicide when he was 15 and I was 12. I didn't know anything. Nobody knew. My grandparents didn't know.

ESS: *How did you learn about it?*

SIS: When I was 23 I was about to be in graduate school, and I moved back home. I broke up with a boyfriend, and I moved back home to my mom's house, and I was going to start graduate school. Anyway, I moved into the big room which used to be Arthur's room. So I had to clean out everything in the room and was moving things and boxing things up and moving them into other rooms, and one of the things that I was moving was his yearbooks from high school. And, you know, I was just kind of looking through my brother's old school pictures, not thinking it was anything private, just enjoying looking at all the funny things. Anyway, I opened up a yearbook and this paper comes out, and this paper is a letter that he had written to himself one day in high school. It was lunchtime or recess time and he wrote: Here I am again, another lunch with nothing to do, and basically saying how he hates the world, he hates life, all these things, how depressed he was, and how every weekday at lunch he sits there all by himself and sits on the floor and writes these letters and pretends he has something to do so that it doesn't look like he is all alone, to make it look like he is actually busy. And in this letter he sounded so upset and so awful. I knew nothing of this. My brother and I were very close. We used to have this five-call rule, which means I could call him only five times a day; this is how much we talked. And we were so close, but I knew nothing of it; and even hearing how depressed he was in that letter, I had no clue of the reality that was going on. And my mom told me how he had tried to commit suicide when he was fifteen, and she told me some of the history of things, and soon after that I approached my brother because, as I said, we were very close, and I said something to him, and he acknowledged everything to me and started telling me about his depression from then on. But before that, I didn't know. He was my normal brother, he was funny as could be; whenever we were anywhere, he made everybody laugh, and everybody decided he was just so smart. And he worked his tail off; it didn't come naturally to him, he had to work so hard to do well in college, to do well in med school. And he was always at the top, but he had to work really hard, and he succeeded, and I just thought he was an amazing guy and never thought anything about this until I was twenty-three when this paper fell out of his things; and from then on, we would talk about things. He would tell me how depressed he was and how hard it was.

ESS: *Did he give you any clues as to the source of this pain?*

SIS: Well, he basically said there wasn't a source.

ESS: *What lay behind it? What was he in pain about?*

SIS: It wasn't really about anything, it was just the pain. As you said, the dysphoria, I guess, you could say it was that, a terrible feeling inside, this terrible pain, this terrible sadness and pain and lack of feeling happy, a lack of enjoying things. And it wasn't because he thought, well, I don't have friends, and if I have friends, I'll be happy and I won't feel the pain; well, I always wanted to get married and have a family, so maybe if I get married and have a family I'll feel happy; and if I have a good career, and—well, at first I think he thought it was that, I don't have these things in life but once I have them, then I'll feel good and then—obviously, I'm not him, so I don't know. But what it seems to me is that, one by one, as he got these things, he realized this wasn't making him feel out of pain, this wasn't making him happy; and one by one all these things that were supposed to make him happy, weren't.

ESS: *Did he say to you that he felt he wasn't worthy or that he wasn't any good?*

SIS: No, he thought in work that he was failing. In his medical work, he was scared that he could jeopardize someone's life or something like that, but in work everyone else said that he was doing an amazing job. So that was the one thing where he thought he wasn't doing well, where he really was; but in regards to being a good person or a kind person and all that—no, he didn't think he was a bad person. I would talk to him about his depression and what he was feeling, and if there was anything I could do to make him feel better. I believe that when someone is suicidal, you try and get them help, and so I'd talk to him, and when he was feeling suicidal, I would ask him if he had a plan; and he said to me that he knew way too much. He said, I'm the doctor, I've done my psych rotation. I know everything there is to know.

ESS: *Did he say, in effect, get off my case?*

SIS: He said it, not in a mean way, but in a way: Listen, there is nothing anyone can do to help me. If you want to try and see if I am suicidal, to put me somewhere to try and get me help, you can't. You can't, because I'm too smart for that; and you can try and put me somewhere, but all it would do is make me pissed off at you, because they can't help me. And if you put me somewhere, I know all of the right things to say, and I'll say what they need to hear, and they'll let me go, and it won't be any help, and I'll just be mad at you for doing what you did.

ESS: *When his death actually occurred, were you surprised?*

SIS: Yes—and the way I found out was awful. I was at my house, my apartment, and I was getting ready, I was supposed to go to my roommate's birthday party, my very good friend. And I received this phone call from the police saying, Are you home, stay home, we'll have to talk to you. And I didn't think about Arthur at all. What I thought about then was, because I had this psycho person who was in love with this guy who I had dated, and she was stalking me and calling me and disconnecting my phone, and she did all these crazy things, and I thought it was about her, and I was scared almost for my life, thinking, well, am I safe in here? And I locked all my doors, and I was scared because I thought it was about her. And then my boyfriend, who is now my fiancé, said to me: Are you sure that was the police that called you? You need to make sure because, God forbid, if it's she who called to make sure you are staying home and she was going to come to your home, she knows where you live, and, God forbid, she's going do something. You need to call the police station and make sure that they honestly called you and she is not pretending she is the police and asking you to stay home. So I called the police station, and I was on hold for a very long time. By this time, my best friend had come over, because we were worried that this woman was trying to do something to me; so she came over to be there and comfort me and be there with me. And I'm still waiting on the phone for about half an hour, and this stupid person at the police station says to me: Do you know somebody that lives on Pine Road? And that's all she had to say. I nearly fell to the floor, and I just said to my friend that my brother had killed himself. That's all she said, and I just knew that Arthur had killed himself. I knew, I immediately knew.

ESS: *You believe now that he was star-crossed?*

SIS: I do, I really do. So many times, after Arthur died, my oldest brother or Arthur's friend would talk about, if we could have done this, if we would have done that—it drives me crazy when they do that.

ESS: *What were some of those things?*

SIS: It wasn't really anything. His friend used to live with Arthur for a period of about six months, and after he moved out, about six months later, is when Arthur committed suicide. So he said, if only he hadn't moved out. That was one of the "ifs." I don't believe in any of them. You asked if [I think] the suicide was inevitable. For lack of a better word, yes, I do, because I feel like we all tried so many things. Arthur was in so many different therapies, tried so many different medications. His best friend, you know, as Arthur said, ratted on him, and when he, years ago, knew Arthur was suicidal, he called his father, not knowing what to do, and said, What do I do? and basically they told Arthur's medical school, they tried to get Arthur help, and Arthur stopped talking to his best friend for months, saying, How dare you do this to me, it's not helping me, and I just, I feel like anything we would have done to help him would have been a temporary help because it was this pain that was inside him that was so strong that, as he described it, it was as if someone was hammering nails into him every second into every part of his body.

ESS: *These were his words?*

SIS: Yes, in one of his letters.

ESS: *He saw a therapist for some years? What's your take on him? Did he sustain him?*

SIS: I don't know. I know a lot of my family thinks he didn't do enough. I don't know. I don't know what to say. Probably for many years Arthur was not aware of what he was feeling himself, and then—I hate to say this, but the reality is sometimes I don't know what someone can do to help, I don't know, when Arthur was in that state, I don't know what anyone could do to make a difference to him than what we did do. I think we all made a difference in that he lived to 30 years old when he was talking about killing himself when he was 7; so maybe if it weren't for all our help he would have killed himself when he was 10 or 15 or 20. But he kept going through these extra years, that I think that part of that is from all the things we did do and all the help that he did get, the therapy and the psychiatrist and all the medications, all of those things I think prolonged his life. But even one of his psychiatrists, towards the end, said basically that he feels that Arthur was one of that small percent where—with a lot of people, if you try one medication, it helps them; other people you have to try a few, and these help them; others you try a lot, and it helps them; and some people the medication doesn't help, and he believed that that was Arthur.

ESS: *Tell me if you will about two women, his wife and his girlfriend.*

SIS: Okay, his wife. They got married when Arthur was 24. They got married very quickly. They were together for less than a year and got married and were married for about 3 years and got divorced. According to Arthur, they fought the whole time, even right before they got married and even on their honeymoon. And I believe he loved her, but I believe also that Arthur always was searching for something to make him happy. And he was definitely a family man; he had always wanted a family, and I think that part of him inside said, if I have a family, then I'll be happy. And he met her, and I believe he was happy for a little while being with her, but then they got married, and I think that inside he realized that this isn't the thing that's making my life out of pain, which I thought it would be;

and I don't think the marriage was very good at all. He said the whole time they fought and things weren't right.

ESS: *Do you think he had a goal of perfection in his own mind? Did you have a presentiment of how things were going to go?*

SIS: Not a clue. I thought they were so happy, and I was so happy for them, and he looked so in love and you could even see that in the pictures of him on that day, he looked really happy; and I think part of it also is, the whole time I always see Arthur as having two paths in life: one was his path of, I'm going to become a doctor and get married and have a good practice and do this and have my family and everything he was going to do, always looking for the future; and at the same time, I'm in pain, I can't take it, I've got to kill myself, I'm in pain, I can't take it, I've got to kill myself. And there were really two separate things, because on the very day he killed himself he had lunch with my father. He asked my father for money. He said Dad, I just had to pay all my taxes and I don't have much money left, can I have 500 dollars to help me through the month? And my dad said he was going to go home and write him a check and send it in the mail. That wasn't a trick on Arthur's part. There is no way in the world that he was trying to trick my father, but I think part of him wanted to go on.

ESS: *Was part of him not talking to the other part?*

SIS: I don't know about that. I don't know, but I feel as though there were those two parts, and he wanted both to be right. He wanted to live; I don't believe he wanted to die, he wanted to live, but he's in pain, and he doesn't want this pain anymore. And the same thing, that day he had spent time with his best friend whose little disposable camera he had, and he said, I'll give it to you during the week. And, again, there is no way in the world that Arthur was just lying to him. He meant, "I'll give it to you in a couple of days when I see you." He had every intention of seeing him, he obviously had every intention of using my dad's money to help him pay his rent for the month, but at the same time at certain times he just couldn't take it any more, he just couldn't deal with it anymore.

ESS: *Please say something about his girlfriend.*

SIS: She was his love. He loved her so much, and I think they had something really special, and they both loved each other so much, but I think the depression ruined their relationship. She was there for him and did everything she could for him—beyond even when they had broken up for a long time, she would still be there for him and do for him whatever she could. But I think that seeing her life and her future, she could only take so much, as opposed to putting herself totally in there, saying this is the life I'm going to live for the rest of my life; but at the same time, it wasn't like she didn't want it and broke off with him. He broke off with her. He broke up with her time and time again And I think again it's the same thing: He wanted to be happy and then was so happy and then couldn't be happy and was happy and couldn't be, and nothing made him happy. And so he'd be with her and break up with her and then wanted to get back together, and even in one of his letters he wrote—because he called her that very night, he called her; they had been broken up for over a year at this point, but she still, if things could have been right with Arthur, I think if he wouldn't have been depressed, she would have married him, and I know she'll always love him very very much. But I know that Arthur was her love, and that very night he called her. And he even wrote in one of his letters—I can't remember the exact words—something to the effect of, even if we would have gotten back together, don't feel bad, don't think that would have saved me, because I know, come another day or a few weeks or months, I wouldn't have been happy and would have done that same cycle and hurt you over again and broken up with you over again and gone through the same thing over and over again. So it's like part of him really understood everything, too. I want us to be back together again and say that's going to save me, but at the same time I know that I'll just do this over again, and I'll just break up with you again and say you're not good for me, and break up with you again and be miserable again and just do it all over again.

ESS: *Tell me something about yourself as a survivor. Where are you in life, what is your own future?*

SIS: I just turned 30. I have my master's in social work. I work mostly with elderly people, doing whatever I can to help them, and I absolutely love my job and it's wonderful. I have a fiancé who is wonderful, and I have great friends and a great family, and I have all those great things, but I miss my brother so much, it just hurts so much, he was one of my best friends, and he was so outstanding. I feel like I don't really understand everything. We were so close, and he was my big brother, and whenever I had big decisions to make, his opinion mattered more than anyone else's. It was like—he was almost like a father figure but at the same time like a really good friend. He'd come to me about friends, and about girls, and all these things, and we'd always help each other and talk about everything, but the last year and a half of his life, he really pulled away; and he would always say because he was busy, he had crazy hours and was always tired and didn't have time for so much else, and he would always just say I'm working, I'm so exhausted. And, also, sometimes he would say I'm depressed, I'm having a bad day, you know, he would say that, too. So for the past year and a half before he died, he wasn't around so much. I guess my point in all of this is that the year and a half before he died, he already was doing so many things separate from us and already wasn't at a lot of our family functions and things like that; and I would call him and cry to him already while he was alive. I'd say Arthur, I miss you, I want to hang out, can I come over; and already I was crying when he was alive, and so I feel now that part of me doesn't really believe he's dead and that some part of me won't ever really believe it, because I'm used to him being there and yet not being there at the same time, while he was alive, that he is just studying or working or at home sleeping and he's not dead; he's just busy being himself. But then the other part of me hurts so much that I just, I miss him so much. It's something so hard to comprehend. And it's hard for me to understand that my brother is really dead and I will never talk to him again, and that's forever.

CONSULTATION BY
JOHN T. MALTSBERGER, M.D.

John T. Maltsberger was born into a Southwest Texas ranching family in 1933. He graduated from Princeton University in 1955 and from the Harvard Medical School in 1959. He trained in psychiatry at the Massachusetts Mental Health Center under Elvin Semrad, completed psychoanalytic training at the Boston Psychoanalytic Institute, and has been engaged in teaching medical students and residents for more than forty years. He is a past president of the American Association of Suicidology, which awarded him the Dublin award in 1994, and secretary of the board of the American Foundation for Suicide Prevention. At the Harvard Medical School, he is associate clinical professor of psychiatry. Among many papers and book chapters, he wrote Suicide Risk: The Formulation of Clinical Judgment *(1986),* Assessment and Prediction of Suicide *(1992), and* The Treatment of Suicidal People *(1994).*

You can read in the Book of Judges about an ancient general named Sisera, who could gain no advantage in battle: Try as he might, he was on the wrong side; God was against him, and he was doomed to perish before he ever started to fight. (It was Sisera who died when Jael drove a tent peg into his temple.) Deborah, the prophetess, sang of him:

> From heaven fought the stars,
> from their courses they fought
> against Sisera.[1]

[1]Judg. 20.

The ancient astrologers taught that the fates of men and nations were written in their stars, and echoes of this belief are still heard in the contemporary metaphor that describes people or enterprises as "star-crossed," or under a malign and inexorable influence, the influence of a dark star. In several places in this book, Professor Shneidman describes the young man of whom we write as "star-crossed." Like accursed Orestes, who fled the furies across land and sea, the protagonist of this book, a young physician-attorney named Arthur, was pursued across his life by inexorable recurring mental anguish. Try as he might, there was no escaping it, until in desperation he killed himself. The ancients recognized those who seemed predestined to destruction and figured them as accursed by the gods, pursued by furies, or, in later times, as possessed by demons. More recently, psychoanalysts discerned the operation of murderous introjects taking possession of the minds of intractably suicidal persons. The up-to-date among us today attribute such evil mental dooms to biology. Those closest to Arthur noticed his relentless march toward suicide that plainly began in his childhood—a march from which no therapy, no pill, no work, no pleasure, and no happiness could long deflect him—and conclude together, as though in a Sophoclean chorus, that it was biology that did it.

It is, of course, disordered biology that kills everybody in the long run—disorders of heart, lungs, gut, or what have you will get us, every one. Disordered brain biology assuredly has its part to play in some deaths, including suicide. But morbid wrong neural connections in the brain or disordered neurotransmitter systems are not the immediate cause of such suicides as this, though assuredly they are more remote and, sometimes, essential causes. The immediate, proximate cause of the suicide we have at hand was ineluctable, unendurable anguish. When no succor comes, the desperate sufferer turns to death for the only possible relief. Shneidman (1993) chooses to call mental anguish "psychache."

If desperate, inescapable, recurring anguish was Arthur's curse, that thing which immediately killed him, where did it come from? What causes can we infer that lay behind the immediate cause?

Something was seriously wrong from early childhood. Arthur's mother and the psychotherapist who saw him as a little boy describe uncontrollable rages and emotional storms; these began by the age of 2 and lasted into latency. He would run through the house with a baseball bat smashing things. He would bite his mother, hit, scream. He seemed beyond comforting. His speech development was delayed. He knocked his kindergarten teacher's glasses off. He was troublesome and disruptive in school. By the third grade, he was "absolutely horrible." There were food peculiarities and intolerances. There was a learning disability. Only later was it discovered that he was unable normally to process auditory information. Something was clearly wrong with the way his brain worked, and we know that children with this kind of social difficulty are particularly vulnerable to major mental illness, including schizophrenia, in adolescence and young adulthood (Hollis, 2003).

We know that the brains of patients with suicidal depression differ from those of normal individuals and that these differences can be demonstrated by neuromagnetic resonant imaging devices (Stoff & Mann, 1997). But the causes of early childhood brain abnormalities that later contribute to affective disorders (and suicide) are obscure. Certainly genetic factors seem likely. We know that Arthur's mother was depressed herself, that there was depression in her forebears. But the brain-injurious effects of viral infections during pregnancy and of difficult labor and delivery are still under investigation. Anoxia at the time of birth can make for future trouble (Neugebauer & Reuss, 1998).

Whatever the biology, our patient seems to have been born with a brain that predisposed him to overarousal and emotional extremes, especially rages, that made it difficult for him to relate to his mother and his teachers. He seemed unable to take comfort and soothing from others in the ordinary way that children do. He repelled others from him. Anyone would have found Arthur repellent, however sweet and winning he could be sometimes. His mother was literally driven to distraction, and the teachers wanted to get him out of the classroom and send him home early.

Many children are born irritable and high-strung, but, given ameliorative circumstances, can in the course of development learn to moderate their moods and quiet themselves down. To some extent, all children must address this task if they are to make it into successful adulthood; all of us as little children are subject to anxieties and other fits of feeling. In normal development, the child takes in quieting, comforting influences from the adults around him and learns how to calm himself down. Successful development of this sort requires, however, that the adults in the infantile milieu have the capacity and the persevering willingness to help a toddler master himself and his inner storms. Not every child is blessed in this way. Often enough, children with stormy, restless temperaments are the offspring of parents with similar temperaments. Further, the temperament of the child must be such so that he does not drive away adults who might otherwise help him grow up. Arthur's wild childhood temperament was extreme. He did not make attachments to adults easily, it would seem, and did many things to upset them and make it difficult for them to succor him in a quiet and comforting way. He was an upsetting child and, to some extent, must have spoiled his own chances for getting essential help from the outside.

Furthermore, though the brains of infants and children are remarkably plastic and capable of great adaptation and adjustment, they are not unlimited in this respect. Maybe Arthur was too extreme in basic neurological organization to make good use of that which was offered him.

In adolescence, Arthur's tantrums and rages slowly appeared to have turned around, no longer taking the outer world, but the patient himself, as their target. As a small boy, he raged against his mother because she did not offer him perfectly what he wanted. As a man, he scorned himself because he was not perfect. Though he was to reject others in his adult life because he could find insufficient comfort in them, he began to reject himself, too. In short, he became depressed. Furthermore, the depression had a strong narcissistic color. Arthur was fastidious about what he would accept from others, and fastidious about what he would accept in himself. *Aut Caesar, aut nihil*—either Caesar or nothing—was to some extent his motto. No woman was beautiful enough or good enough, no achievement of his own sufficiently perfect. Short of perfection, he was miserable, miserably depressed.

The tragedy of the story is plain: Arthur went through life looking for something, anything, from outside himself, to help moderate his intolerable feelings—but to be acceptable, it had to be perfect. As a child, he flew into rages and rejected his mother because she did not (could not) help him with his distress. He repeated this pattern with a young wife, with a girlfriend, and with others when he grew to manhood. His friendship with another man was insufficient. His work was not enough to quiet his pain, though he tried very hard at it. Psychotherapy appears to have helped somewhat at various times in his life, but not enough to make the critical difference.

Arthur never achieved an essential developmental task—to accept the necessary limitations of life. Life can never be perfect. Maybe perfect comforting is attainable in early infancy, but never later, certainly not in adulthood. Successful adulthood demands that one must passively endure disappointment over and over again, and, accepting "second best," get on with what one can have. Maturity demands that one must accept passive suffering without flying into rages against life or against one's body.

Painful disappointments that cannot be changed must be endured. This sad truth is one that Arthur never learned, yet it is a fundamental rule of life. The boy who is too small and too uncoordinated to become a fine athlete must endure his fate. The man who has had too many losses and from whom old age steals health must endure his lot or otherwise fly into fruitless narcissistic rage and depression. The capacity to renounce an omnipotent, perfect self-image and to accept the necessary limitations of reality are decisive for containing depression. Closely related to these is the capacity to forgive others for their failings and to love them anyway. Those whose relations to others are highly ambivalent and whose self-esteem depends too much on high performance or excessive gratification are highly vulnerable (Zetzel, 1965). Arthur was such a person.

There were some trials with psychopharmacy. There is a suggestion that he abandoned this avenue as a source of help in the last months of his life, although it does not appear that the pharmacopoeia had been by any means exhausted; there were no trials, for instance, of monoamine oxidase inhibitors. Neither is it clear that he had adequate doses for an adequate period of time of venlafaxine (Effexor), fluoxetine (Prozac), or citalopram (Celexa). If he could not tolerate lithium salts, other mood-stabilizing drugs *might* have helped. Electroconvulsive treatment might have made a difference, although it would not, I think, have been a permanent solution. There are those who would have advised a neurosurgical approach, though I have known patients who believed suicide a better option, in spite of the good results reported (Hodgkiss, 1994). (I have met some clinicians who think that, too.) Such operations are difficult to arrange in the United States, easier in Canada and the United Kingdom; and they do not turn those who receive them into lobotomized cabbages. Maybe this was an avenue Arthur might have pursued had it been offered him. He said he was open to electroconvulsive treatment at one point.

Given Arthur's temperament, I suspect he might have been a difficult patient to treat with drugs: He was quick to reject and very strong minded. Psychotherapy would have been difficult, too, because the angry, rejecting child with the baseball bat, fighting and biting, was always in the background. Overtly or covertly, he would hate the therapist in due time for failing to produce relief from the anguish. If the hate remained hidden, the therapist might be lulled into agreeing to premature interruption. Arthur never came to terms with his narcissistic rage in the treatment described in the protocols. Figuratively speaking, no doctor could have gone far with Arthur unless he were prepared to lay hold of his patient and to hang on to him with great emotional tenacity for a long time. Whether Arthur would have permitted a more intense treatment is difficult to know.

My experience with patients like Arthur makes me mistrust split therapies, with one person in charge of drug prescription and another in charge of the psychotherapy. Much can get lost in trios that does not escape a therapeutic duet. I see nothing in the protocols that suggests that the split treatment resulted in the ultimate suicide that happened here; however, they do in some.

INTERVIEW WITH THE PAL

ESS: *You are designated as Arthur's best friend and pal. Tell me a little about yourself.*

PAL: I'm single. I have a girlfriend. I have an MBA, and I work in marketing.

ESS: *Now please tell me about Arthur, when you met him and how long you knew him, and what kind of fellow he was.*

PAL: I met him in summer camp, we were cocounselors. For the year or two that we were counselors, we were friends, but we weren't actually that close. And then we went to the university together. We were freshmen there together, and I didn't know anybody, and I remember calling him, saying, "Hey, I'm coming; let's hang out, please." And so we became very close very quickly once college started. I remember going through a lot of change together; that's when we started investing in an emotional relationship, something that was real. And it gradually just got stronger and stronger, continued getting stronger and stronger, and there was some acknowledgment maybe when we would talk about it—maybe ten years ago—that maybe we truly were best friends; and I felt comfortable with him. It's hard to explain; it's a feeling that you can do whatever you want in front of the person, that was it; and vice versa. And we both felt that way. I moved here right after college, so we've always been around for each other. It's hard to describe Arthur: He was unique and very talented in many ways; he was very likeable; a very likeable, easy person; all my friends liked him. He was tough and stubborn and really liked to engage and get into issues and debate, but in a very nonabrasive, nonthreatening way. He was a sweet guy. I mean he was just a really sweet guy. He was fun, he liked to go out; at least earlier on, he liked to go out, back in college. Later on, as he became more depressed, he would not go out as much. I'd invite him out. I didn't know anything about his depression actually until probably five years ago. He was in a marriage, and he got divorced. I would always ask him, "How is the marriage going?" and he'd always say, "It's okay. Marriage is tough." And then one day we were driving, and he pulled me over and he just started crying and told me how bad his marriage was, and then—oh, and we got closer, and that was another stage, because he was embarrassed. He always said, "Marriage is a proclamation to everybody, and I'm failing at this." And he was embarrassed to tell me about it, felt like a failure. And then, once he was able to communicate how bad his relationship was, that, I think, allowed him to then reveal his depression for the first time. Like how depressed he was I had no idea. I didn't know that he had an incident when he was 15. I didn't know about that until about five years ago. And so that brought it to a different level—I mean, I could just continue talking about different things. I want to stick to the question, What is Arthur like?

ESS: *Were there any crazy elements in his behavior?*

PAL: Oh, yeah.

ESS: *A psychotic element?*

PAL: I don't think he was psychotic; neurotic.

ESS: *Did he ever behave as though he were responding to voices?*

PAL: No, that's why it never got to the psychosis level. I mean, he would respond to impulses. I didn't think of it at the time, I thought of him as Arthur. I guess when I use the word "crazy" it's more like "wacko," like he's just a weird guy, not crazy-psychotic; there is a difference to me. I just thought Arthur was unique, and he was just like a weird, cool, crazy guy—because he would just do stuff like that, and he was a little socially awkward at times yet could also be totally charming. He was fairly happy being a doctor. And he was happy being a lawyer. I imagine that he was very good because he was compassionate. He compartmentalized. Somehow he got it together, although he did get into some disciplinary trouble with administrators; they called him "Controversy," that was his nickname. But that was Arthur, that was stirring the pot. Arthur would want to know: "Why is the system like this, why don't we do this?" And it would get him into trouble because he certainly wasn't a conformist, by any means. Yet, with the patients or clients, I don't think he would do anything wacko or crazy in that context. I think he treated that with special care, and he was very nurturing; and that's part of the weird dichotomy. He would take, I mean, he had some bottles of stuff, like, besides antidepressants. One night—and I let him do whatever he wanted—one night he had some stuff from the hospital, and he shot himself up with Demerol or something, I'm not really sure what it was, but what could I do? I was just there for him, and I knew that he really didn't have any other close relationships to talk to.

ESS: *Did you see him as a needful person?*

PAL: Well, all at the same time entirely needy and at the same time, like, I don't need you, I don't need anybody.

ESS: *Including the need for autonomy?*

PAL: Including the need for autonomy. There were times when he would call me, crying, and ask me to come over. But more, I would have to ask him, "Do you want me to come over?" "Yeah, that would be cool." He didn't want to ask me all the time. He felt, again, embarrassed. I had to be like, "Arthur, I should come over." "Yeah, that would be cool, I could use company."

ESS: *We can ask some more specific questions. What do you mean, how bad the marriage was, what was bad specifically? Tell me more.*

PAL: They did fight a lot. I think that he met her and they were engaged after eight weeks, and Arthur was the kind of guy—he felt like he needed to have the marriage and to have certain things in his life, and I think he didn't really know her.

ESS: *What, for appearance' sake?*

PAL: I think in his own mind he knew he was very depressed; and I think this may have been a way for him to have stuff and things that could maybe take that away. Maybe if he had that, he wouldn't feel as bad. I think he went to medical school right after college. His father was a doctor, and he felt he had to have a certain professional responsibility and being an adult; when he expounded on his relationship, he didn't get into it so much with her other than the fact that he felt like he didn't know her and that she had her own issues, that he couldn't communicate with her. I mean, most things come down to communication. I didn't see the two of them together so much because, during that time [that] the relationship was bad, he didn't want me there with the two of them. He would come out and meet me separately, or he'd invite me over when she wasn't there because he didn't want me around then, so I therefore did not actually see it or have great insight into their relationship. But I think, in retrospect, his clinical depression played a role, had to have played a role in the demise of that relationship.

ESS: *What do you understand when you say "clinical depression"?*

PAL: Clinical depression? The chemistry in the brain is off, it's actually, I think, treatable by drugs. Clinical depression, organic, is something that's genetic somewhat or something you need to treat as a cancer. It's not a situational depression, it's something that—as he said, he was "dealt a bad hand." That is, he was dealt the hand of clinical depression.

ESS: *Genetically?*

PAL: Genetically. He had such a self-awareness about his situation. It scared me. To be so self-aware, and when you have that condition, is a tough combination.

ESS: *What do you think his devils were? What was he so in pain about?*

PAL: Arthur would get on a level sometime when I would say: "Why are you unhappy, what does the pain feel like, where does the pain come from?" and he would say things like, "Life just doesn't mean much to me, it's boring, I don't see the point"; he would say general philosophical, theoretical things: "I don't understand what the point is," and it would always come out, we would end up talking about how he didn't have any relationships going on, and that was always sort of a big focus. But I think the bigger, deeper thing with him was—what I don't understand, because we would have these discussions and he would sigh and say, "I'm bored all the time, I don't know what to do."

ESS: *And how did you react to that? Did you see that as a challenge to try to bring him back to life, to cheer him up and so on?*

PAL: I tried to. I saw it as a challenge, but I also thought, from how he was talking, that it would be difficult to do that because he was talking in terms that I kind of couldn't relate to. It's hard to argue against something like that: What's the point of living. Sometimes it's hard to counter with A, B, C, and D—you can have kids, you can become a professional, so—"Well, that doesn't mean anything to me"; when you say that, I took it as, it was a paradigm shift. Once he started talking to me like that, I said, Okay, he's dealing in a different reality; I'm going to be there for him, but there isn't really much I can do without professional help.

ESS: *Did you think that he was a kind of born pessimist?*

PAL: No, I don't think he was a born pessimist. I mean because he changed when we were in college; he was excited about things to me; he was different; I believe that he changed and got worse, and he would look forward to things and to going out; he was excited about being in a relationship. We went river rafting together. He wanted to take a weekend trip, and he was excited about that, and he'd reminisce about that. So he was optimistic, yet, I guess, as he got deeper into the pessimism, which is a by-product of deeper stuff going on, he changed. But at the same time I say he changed, it's harder for me to have any objectivity about his condition, because I was with him so much. Not only were we best friends emotionally, psychologically; in practical terms we were best friends, because we hung out together. I saw him quite a bit, so it's very hard for me to step back and say, here is A, here is B. Obviously, in retrospect, the last couple of months were pretty bad.

ESS: *You are saying, you are describing a fellow who habitually distorted the world in this pessimistic, dysphoric, dark-colored way. Are you saying that this began after college? And do you have hints other than genetic predisposition as to where that might have come from, psychologically?*

PAL: His parents were divorced when he was eight, I mean, it's hard for me to know what that meant to him.

ESS: *What are you implying?*

PAL: I certainly think there was trauma there. We did talk about it a little bit but not so much, but I know he was 8 years old, and, of course, I didn't know him until he was 16, so this is all before me.

ESS: *Did he then sort of form a paradigm of the world that one couldn't trust the world?*

PAL: I think somewhat. He had a strained relationship with his mother. I would go over there and he—it was very tough to see the two of them together. He was tough on his mom, and he had a hard time dealing with his parents, relationship-wise.

ESS: *Please say more about that. Apparently, in his lifetime, you were one of the few people that he really trusted.*

PAL: Yeah, he felt as not being in a family. My personality is very easygoing, and I think he always just felt comfortable telling me whatever, and he knew that I wouldn't betray his trust.

ESS: *And you didn't have an agenda for him.*

PAL: No. He would talk to me a little bit about his parents; his not really having much respect for his father; he would say it in terms of very black and white. I remember we were at a bookstore, and he said, "You know what, I'm going to stop talking to my dad; I don't have a need to talk to my dad. To me, I don't get anything out of that, and I'm gonna stop talking to him." And then his mother he was closer to; therefore, he was more strained. He had much more invested with his mother; therefore, he would lash out at her, because, I think, he felt his mother could understand his pain a little more and therefore he pushed her away, I think. He wasn't as uncomplimentary about her as he was about his dad, actually. The typical: She nags me, she doesn't give me space, very typical things. I don't think, he never revealed to me the depth, the deep-rooted psychological stuff going on with his mother; this is just what I'm thinking it was.

ESS: *But you're implying that there was something deeper.*

PAL: I think a similar pathology, in a way, with his mother. Again, I'm just thinking she could maybe understand his pain, or he was embarrassed in front of his mother a little bit more. I don't know that—just getting back to the general context of what I was answering, you were saying, besides genetics—I don't know, we can talk about all of those things—I think it's a clinical thing, I mean it doesn't matter really, well, it does matter, contributing to it. We had a conversation about six months before he died, and I said, "Arthur, you know, we're going to be best friends." Because I loved him, he was my first best friend. He made me open myself up more emotionally, he was the first person, the first sort of male friend, non-girl-friend. And so we had this conversation; I said, "You know, we're going to know each other for the rest of our lives," and he said, "Well, you never know, though, because I could move away, you never know, I could marry someone you don't like." I couldn't believe, it just struck me as peculiar.

ESS: *So he had a dark-side answer for almost everything.*

PAL: That was clearly a dark-side answer. I'm saying we are going to know each other for the rest of our lives because we are best friends, assuming we're going to die naturally.

ESS: *And he responded pessimistically, like, that's not certain.*

PAL: Right. I think certainly he became more and more pessimistic, because when life doesn't matter, the little things in it are meaningless. He was always looking for deeper meaning in everything. I mean, if there is this cable, he would want to know where it came from, I mean just anything. He would get into things.

ESS: *It has a history, but that is a digression.*

PAL: He did this for me. The day he died, I saw him that Sunday, I hung out with him, and there was a problem with my car alarm, and he drilled this hole that Sunday. And when he left that morning he said, "Ta ta."

ESS: *What time was this?*

PAL: About eleven o'clock in the morning.

ESS: *Did he die that day?*

PAL: That night, that night; we hung out that day.

ESS: *He wrote a note.*

PAL: Well, he started writing his note Friday night, I believe, and then he finished it Sunday night.

ESS: *On Sunday morning, there seemed no intimation of his suicidal intent. I take it that you were totally surprised by his suicide.*

PAL: Shocking, shocking. Given everything I knew about him. Given the fact that we talked about suicide. Given knowing about his depression. Given his disassociation with life, given all of that—shocking.

ESS: *Do you feel he kept secrets from you? Mainly, the nature of the demons that he had?*

PAL: Yes. I don't think he felt he could communicate them. I think it was very hard for him, and/or he didn't want to share because I couldn't understand.

ESS: *Didn't want to burden you?*

PAL: Yeah, that was part of it, too, the stigma. For Arthur, it was very tough, because he was truly unique. He could compartmentalize his life, he had his professional side, he could hang out with me. He could compartmentalize completely, and he wanted to be a trouper and wanted to try and go out and give to me and not be a burden. I mean, it must have [been] very difficult having been weighted down by the demons.

ESS: *The question in the air is: Do you think he might have been saved? If so, how and by whom?*

PAL: I have to say I think he might have been saved—the answer to that is yes, he could have, he might have been saved. I don't know if he could have been saved, I don't know—there is a certain percentage of people who never get better. If he had gotten into this one clerkship. If he had, maybe, gotten back into a relationship, he might have started to get to a place where he was more stable and then maybe he would have been more willing to try more medications or treatments. It would have gotten him to a place where he could have possibly given it one more crack, two more cracks. That being said, he tried for years and years of medication. Who could have saved him? I mean, I tried. I intervened at one point and I called—one of the first times he told me about everything—I called my father, and he intervened and got Arthur on a program, and Arthur and I didn't speak for months after that. He was so upset that I intervened and I messed up everything and I was all he had and how could I do that; and that put a tremendous strain on the relationship, like big time, for a while. But I wanted to do something. I would have hoped that that could have saved him. Maybe if that hadn't happened, he may have done it sooner, but it doesn't matter; it may have prolonged it. It seems like everything with Arthur was just a prolonging of the inevitable. It seems like his deep-seated, deep-rooted thing, I mean that was just so deep that if medication doesn't work for it, what else can you do? But I was totally shocked, totally shocked. You simply cannot understand the act. How can you understand the act? I can't understand the act.

CONSULTATION BY RONALD MARIS, Ph.D.

Professor Maris is the professional sociologist in this roundtable of experts. For years he has been director of the Suicide Center at the University of South Carolina, and currently he is distinguished professor emeritus (in psychiatry and sociology) at that university. He was born in 1936. He attended the University of Illinois (where he was a National Science Foundation Fellow), and he has done graduate work in Philadelphia, at Harvard, and at Johns Hopkins. For 15 years he was editor of the journal Suicide and Life-Threatening Behavior. *He is the author or editor of several books, including* Social Forces in Urban Suicide *(1969) and* Pathways to Suicide *(1981). He is one of the outstanding living scholars of suicidology.*

Death and suicide can be postponed but not prevented. "We've all got it coming," as Clint Eastwood reminds us in *Unforgiven*. Like most people who commit suicide, Arthur was done in prematurely by a variety of developmental, biological, and interactive bad luck.

First, notably and distinctively, Arthur "raged." He was unusually combative (says his psychotherapist: "One of the angriest children I have known"). It is tempting here to oversimplify and see Arthur's incipient self-destruction as rooted in narcissistic rage at the failure of his mother to love him well enough early on (Spitz, Bowlby). Arthur told his wife, "my parents never let me love them." Arthur's therapist points to Arthur's mother as a special target of his anger. Later on, this lack of basic trust in mother (Jung) seems to transfer to a series of doomed female relationships with wife and girlfriend.

Yet, to argue that Arthur was done in by a self-preoccupied, needy mother is like arguing that Sylvia Plath was a "man hater." In fact, Arthur raged at the world. He fought his older brother, his father, his pal, his teachers and schoolmates, any people who would befriend him; at age 5, he punched his own therapist in the groin. In fact, Arthur raged at life itself, at his pitiful human condition. Life itself was intolerably painful (like "hammered nails in every inch of my body," or like "lying on a bed of needles").

Wherever this rage came from (of course, it could be biologically based, too), eventually anger and rage did their part to doom Arthur. As Menninger tells us, rage tends to turn back on oneself. People like Arthur tend to end up trying to kill the world, or at least their world.

Developmentally, Arthur and most suicides I have known have what I call a "suicidal career" (Maris, 1981). I wrote: "Suicidal decisions develop over time and against certain psychological and genetic or biological backdrops, they are never explained completely by acute situational factors." Arthur had been suffering a long time (at least 25 years) and had multiple suicidogenic forces in his life. His wife contends that his suicidal vulnerability was a "lifelong pattern."

Suicidal careers imply repetition of risk and failure of protective factors. In a sense, what happened on the Sunday Arthur killed himself was not especially important (such as having had lunch with his father, being separated from his girlfriend, not being in therapy, etc.). His psychiatrist says he knew Arthur would commit suicide "someday." Arthur's fragile coping crumbled with *repeated* depressive episodes, *repeated* psychic pain, *repeated* interpersonal failures and disappointments, and *repeated* suicide ideation and suicide attempts. His suicide risk gradually summated until a pain and suicide threshold was nondramatically (if not this day, then some other) breached.

Second, Arthur probably had a biologically based, recalcitrant, nonresponsive major depression (note that all of Arthur's suicidogenic forces overlap and interact). To say Arthur fell "doomed from the womb" is an exaggeration, but something close to that happened. His anhedonia was startling, present very early on, and not especially responsive to antidepressant medications (viz., to Effexor, Wellbutrin, Prozac, lithium). Arthur was one of those among us who have too little "joy juice" (Kramer, 1993).

Arthur's psychiatrist proclaimed: "I was *positive*" [emphasis added] [that] "someday he was going to commit suicide . . . his depression was a biological curse." Sure, Arthur could have been forcibly hospitalized and given electroconvulsive therapy (ECT; his psychiatrist considered this), but to what end? Would it be just postponing his suicidal death and prolonging his exquisite suffering? Perhaps. But, to be fair, some major depressions relent, ameliorate, burn down, or even out over time. Maybe Arthur just needed someone to "buy time" for him?

Note that Arthur's being a physician, clever, and bright operated against his even getting proper treatment. Who helps the helpers? I am reminded of Ernest Hemingway's avoiding proper treatment at the Mayo Clinic for his major depression by charming his doctors, wearing green surgical scrubs, and eating lunch with them in the doctors' dining room; in short, refusing to be a patient.

Often violent, self-destructive people like Arthur have a "serotonergic dysfunction" (especially low brain 5-HT and 5-HIAA). Brown, Linnoia, and Goodwin (1992, p. 591) point to serotonergic traits found in animal studies, including impulsivity, disinhibition, sleep difficulties, pain-proneness, conduct disorders, mood volatility, poor peer relationships, and suicidal behaviors (sounds like Arthur to me).

Third, another piece in the puzzle ("enigma") of Arthur's suicidal career was his unreachable, unrealistic, perfectionist expectations of himself and others. Nothing was ever good enough for Arthur (of course, this is often a trait of depressive disorder). This perfectionism resulted in a tortured, virtually impossible existence for him.

Frequently, such high expectations come from mom and/or dad. I found it remarkable that his mom wasn't even mentioned in Arthur's suicide note, and neither did his dad play a prominent role. Arthur's mom was rigid, strict, a little cold, and self-preoccupied (narcissistic). Arthur hardly saw her after his parents divorced. Arthur's father comments that Arthur "raged against his mother's rules."

For Arthur, becoming a medical doctor and then a lawyer, being offered a Supreme Court Justice clerkship, marrying a woman who was a physician, and later having a devoted girlfriend were all not enough ... like a 5-dollar payment on a million-dollar debt. What successes and pleasures Arthur experienced were counterbalanced and even dwarfed by his repeated pain. Reflecting on the platitude that "suicide is a permanent solution to a temporary problem" (in his note), Arthur insists: "life is *not* a temporary problem."

For such would-be suicides as Arthur, nothing is "good enough." Impossible demands are made on oneself and on one's family, profession, and life. Parents are not good enough, siblings are not good enough, careers are not good enough; they are in relentless pursuit of a life that just does not exist in this world.

Fourth, Arthur's suicide was enigmatic in the sense that several features of it were unusual or atypical. To begin with, most adult white male suicides do not even write suicide notes. Only about 15–25% of all suicides (including women) leave *any* note. Certainly they don't leave long (I got tired of reading Arthur's), repeated notes ("dozens of times before," he tells us) and make repeated nonfatal suicide attempts. In my study of thousands of Chicago suicides, almost 90% of all older white males made only *one*, fatal, suicide attempt.

Furthermore, male suicide completers tend to get drunk (why is there no mention of alcohol abuse with Arthur?) and shoot themselves in the head. No guns in Arthur's case. Why not? I developed 15 "predictors" or common traits of suicide (Maris et al., 2000, p. 80). Arthur had only two-thirds of them. In addition to lack of prominent alcohol abuse and not using a gun, there were no suicides in Arthur's family, he was successful at work, and he was not physically ill.

This suggests to me that Arthur's suicide was different or unique in ways that hinted at interventions. He was probably, in fact, ambivalent (not hopeless); he was writing notes to people telling them how awful he felt (why do that if you do not want some response?). And he was using reversible attempt methods.

Fifth, I would be remiss, as the one sociologist reviewing Arthur's case, not to indicate some interactive social forces in his demise. In spite of Arthur's "biological curse" of anhedonia, biology normally is not destiny. Biological misfits are routinely sustained by love and interactive support.

But Arthur had a double sociological whammy. First, his significant "udders" gave sour milk. Second, he rejected sustaining acts of human kindness. To wit:

Mom was cold, strict, and rigid.
Dad was distant and disrespected.
Mom and dad divorced.
Brother was a brilliant competitive bully.
Wife herself was lonely.
Girlfriend came from a family of depressives.

Psychiatrist did not take charge and do what he knew he needed to do (e.g., hospitalization and ECT).

Arthur himself had a fatal interactive flaw: his inability to accept love ("I don't deserve to be happy," "I don't deserve to have a good, attractive woman"). He repeatedly rejected sustaining acts of interpersonal kindness.

Sixth and finally, could Arthur have been saved? His brother and ex-wife say yes. One of his sisters, his girlfriend, his psychotherapist, and his psychiatrist say no. His pal isn't sure. So who's right? You can *always* save people for a while (but no one forever). The pertinent considerations are questions of (1) the costs and (2) their quality of life. In utopias (such as Huxley's *Brave New World*) no properly conditioned citizen is suicidal. Yet, in the Brave New World, no one is free to suffer, to be different, or to be independent. So who would want to live there (if you had a choice)? Kay Jamison (1996) talks about her reluctance to take her lithium (for bipolar disorder) and sacrifice her exquisite manic highs.

There is also involuntary treatment, hospitalization, chemical confinement, straitjackets, suicide-proof environments, 24-hour, 7-day suicide watches, and so forth. But what happens when treatment ends or is not effective? About 30% percent of major depressive disorders do not show a therapeutic response to selective serotonin reuptake inhibitors (SSRIs; certainly Arthur did not). Might ECT have saved Arthur's life? You cannot lock noncriminals up forever. You cannot easily or practically reparent them or rewire their brains. Do we actually want to force people with malignant, nonresponsive depressive disorder to suffer just to please others?

Perhaps if Arthur could have bought some time, the edge would have come off his exquisite psychic pain. Perhaps not. Remember, the standard in life is "good enough." We have come full circle now from my opening comments: Not just Arthur, but none of us, are ever going to get out of this alive. In the meantime, we need to settle for what we have or could get with reasonable effort and a modest genetic endowment. If we cannot do that with some help, then there is always Arthur's resolution.

INTERVIEW WITH
THE EX-WIFE

ESS: *Please tell me about yourself.*

EX-WIFE: I'm a physician, a nephrologist, and I see patients. I'm also a researcher. I do research, and I have some familiarity with an autopsy. You create empirical research, but I do understand the idea of starting out with an open mind and seeing what comes. That you can't start an endeavor such as this with a goal, looking for certain answers, because they don't always come. I do understand that, but intellectually I am interested in whatever it is that you are able to learn. I don't feel that there is really anything in particular that I need to get out of this or to learn in relation to Arthur. I am currently in my fourth year of psychoanalysis since my relationship with Arthur ended. So I feel like I'm getting what I need there. I'm learning about myself, and I'm answering any questions for myself that need to be answered. But I am interested intellectually in your thoughts. I know that you are going to speak to several people, and I'm just interested in what those thoughts would be.

ESS: *You are very special in this process. Tell me more about yourself, and then tell me about Arthur.*

EX-WIFE: It's very complex to describe myself. I think a lot of who I am, I've been discovering over the past 4 years in this psychoanalysis that I have undertaken. I think it's one of the most fascinating and worthwhile endeavors that I've ever done.

Basically, I spent the first 22 years of my life or so, and then I met Arthur. Actually, I met Arthur probably when I was 14, at a summer camp, but nothing really came of it. More time elapsed, and then I remet him when I was in medical school. I was maybe 22 or so. I spent most of my childhood and young adulthood feeling very lonely and sad and not very self-confident. And most people wouldn't be aware of that because on the exterior, I've always earned very high grades, I've always been very successful in the things I undertake. I was a cheerleader in high school, I was on the student body council, I got straight into the college of my choice and the medical school of my choice and so on; but underneath there was something very lonely and troubled. I came to know Arthur, and he was this wonderful thing in my life when we first met. He gave me the feeling that I really made him happy and I really made his life a greater place. And it was a wonderful feeling for me because that was something I never had with my own family growing up. It really filled a hole that I had. So that tells you something about both of us. I'll step back and go backwards from there. My parents emigrated to the United States. They both were born soon after World War II in Austria. My father's mother and father each had their own family, entire family, with children and all, taken into concentration camps, and only his mother and father survived. And they met each other after they were liberated. My grandmother actually walked into a gas chamber, and it was turned on, when the American planes came bombing at liberation. She didn't die. I guess there were too many people for the concentration of gas they were given, so she survived. She met my grandfather. After the war they married. They had my father and a younger sister, who is my aunt, and never spoke again about where they came from or that anyone had perished or they had left anyone behind. And I remember when I was 12, my father lost his mother, the one who had been gassed in the camps, when he was maybe 14. She died of cancer, likely because of this. His father lived; he remained alive until I was approximately 12 years old, and I remember being 12 and going with my father back to New York, where their home was, and I remember him finding these photographs. And it was just recently, in the last couple of decades, that he realized that he wasn't the first child in the family; so there is this whole secret which had never been spoken about. Now I knew that my grandparents had been in a concentration camp because they had the tattoos, the numbers on their arms. They never ever spoke about it. So there is this secret loss.

ESS: *It was understood you were not to point to that and ask about it?*

EX-WIFE: I don't remember, but I know that I don't know what country they came from, and I really know very little about it. I grew up watching my father watch Holocaust movies, and I can remember being very small, like 3 or 4, and seeing footage of Nazi soldiers shooting children, which was very frightening; and I'm now at an age just starting to understand, just quite how broken my family of origin is. I can tell you some more stories on my mother's side. My mother comes from a family with a lot of tragedy. My mother was raised by her grandmother because her parents were new immigrants and worked long hours in a factory. She came home one day and found her grandmother dead. And her parents lied to her and said, "she is not dead, she is sick. She is going to the hospital." But of course she never saw her grandmother again. So again it's the hiding of tragedy.

ESS: *Was it a natural death?*

EX-WIFE: It was a natural death. But, still, for a young girl not to be able to express the loss of the primary caregiver; not to be able to express the terrible loss she must have felt; it must have been very difficult.

ESS: *Do you feel that Arthur had secrets about himself that he never shared with you?*

EX-WIFE: I don't think it was about secrets, but what I do think it was marked by, both of us had some terrible hole inside of us that we didn't understand. I certainly didn't understand it at the time. I'm just getting to know after four years of analysis. But going back, I do think that my relationship with Arthur was characterized by terrible loss—not loss but something terribly missing or wrong inside—and I think both of us were looking for someone to fill that.

ESS: *Can you make the ineffable spoken? Can you verbalize what that hole was for Arthur?*

EX-WIFE: For him, I honestly don't know why, but I can tell you; in retrospect I can look back at him and I can see a lifelong pattern. From what I know of him—I didn't know him when he was small, but he has told me that he had a terrible time in school. He felt terribly alone, and had no friends, a terrible time. And then he came to summer camp and that was one of the years I first met him, and he was extremely happy. He was somewhat popular; he had a lot of friends, and he thought this was what he had been missing. We didn't notice each other at that time. And then, basically, he told me of a whole series of things that came into his life that made him believe that all his pain was going to be better. First it was his school situation, that all his unhappiness must have been because he didn't like the school he went to. But he went to summer camp, and he was very happy, and that gave him the motivation or energy to change schools. So he did change schools, but then he wasn't any happier. Then, I believe, I might be getting these in the wrong order; maybe before that is when his parents got divorced. I think he was younger at that point, he may have been 10, and the divorce was wrong, and that was causing all his pain. I think that he believed that if they got back together, then that would be all better. But that never happened.

Then, he was unhappy. This was when he met me. One of our first conversations was about how unhappy he was because he chose law school instead of medical school. That if he had just chosen medical school, he could be happy. And eventually he went to medical school first. But he caused a huge fight between us because we were engaged. I was already in medical school, and we were going to get married in the near future, and all of a sudden he comes home and he said that there was something he had to do. "I'm applying to medical school." And he started applying throughout the country and outside the country, and I thought: Can't you wait a couple of years, then I'll be done with medical school and I can go with you wherever you need to go. But it was like he was possessed, he just had to do it right away. And his explanation to me was that if he can't be happy inside, the marriage can't be a happy marriage, and he absolutely had to do this. So he did. He applied to medical school, and he was sure that this would solve the problem. And then he was so insecure, he begged me to come and talk with the dean, because I was a student there at the time, to allow him to enter medical school.

ESS: *And you did that?*

EX-WIFE: Yes, and the dean listened to me, but he wasn't going to make any decision based on me. I told Arthur that I had spoken with the dean. I thought it would make him feel better. Then, on his own merit, he got in. He was quite a good student, and he never believed me that he did it on his own merit. And from then on out he always believed that it was I who got him in and that he never deserved it. This made me feel terrible.

ESS: *So you were damned if you did and damned if you didn't?*

EX-WIFE: Yes. He did great in medical school. He got fantastic grades. He is a very intelligent person and very driven and, no matter how well he did, he never believed it was on his own merit. He never believed that he deserved it, that he wasn't a fake, and that he didn't get in because of me.

ESS: *That's the right word, that he "wasn't a fake."*

EX-WIFE: There again, there was this pattern of looking for things that would make him feel better; and he thought that if we got married, that would make him feel better because his parents' divorce made him so upset. His family was broken and not intact. Now that he was getting married, he would have an intact family, and that would make the pain feel better. But still, after he got married, he didn't feel better. I think he must have been terribly disillusioned to find himself in that great degree of pain that he was in. As I was describing before, before we got married he made me feel as if I was the sunshine in his life, that I just made everything all better. And that was really very intoxicating for me because I never had a good relationship with anyone. And then, after we got married, it was as if I made his entire world black.

ESS: *Were there turning points? Could you see the shift in his orientation?*

EX-WIFE: It was pretty much from the day we got married, and it never came back. It never was happy after that. Even on the honeymoon, we would have terrible fights. He would tell me things like, you make me feel like a monster; you push me to hurt you. He never was really a monster, but what he would do was he would really retreat and isolate himself. That was really hard for me.

ESS: *Did he ever physically abuse you? Did he ever hit you?*

EX-WIFE: Never, not once. But he would get really withdrawn, and it would be like five or six days until he would talk to me again. He would really retreat into himself.

ESS: *Can you say what might precipitate something like that?*

EX-WIFE: I would cry. I would need something from him that he wasn't giving, and I would assert that. I remember, we had very different levels of comfort for how clean the house should be. I would come to him and say: "You know I'm not comfortable with things being as messy as they are. I really want you to help," and I would complain. Once he felt criticized or not good enough, he would get very defensive, and we would have terrible fights.

ESS: *Now I want to move to an intimate and taboo topic, your sexual life.*

EX-WIFE: That's an interesting question. What I can tell you, which is not really answering your question exactly, but before we got married he definitely had a sexual interest. We did not have sexual intercourse before we got married. Once we did get married, he seemed to lose the sexual interest somewhat, and it became very distant, and it was mentally disappointing for me. It didn't feel intimate or loving. Once we got married, we didn't have a very active sex life.

ESS: *Here was a fellow who wanted certain things, but the attainment of those things was habitually disappointing to him.*

EX-WIFE: I would agree with that. My guess is that he was always looking to cure some inner pain with outside pain, and he'd get this feverish, he had to do this, and this would fix the pain. But they were always outside things. Getting married, having an intact family, being a physician, being as good at Scrabble as his brother—there is a whole list of things that he attempted to achieve, and he did, but when he got them, the inner pain wasn't gone.

ESS: *Can you think of anything in his life that was an unmitigated triumph and satisfaction for him?*

EX-WIFE: No.

ESS: *Do I dare ask, what about his current girlfriend?*

EX-WIFE: I like her very much.

ESS: *Tell me about that relationship.*

EX-WIFE: That came after me, so I don't know that much. I do know that we went out to lunch with some friends, had a great time, came home saying what a great time we had, and then told me several hours later that he had to end the marriage. It was interesting that Arthur— I'll get there via a circuitous route—that Arthur's times of utmost despair came immediately after happy times. He would cry, and with tears running down his face would tell me that he just couldn't bear how he felt and that he wanted to go far away where no one knew him, and just start over. Which I never understood, because his family always seemed so much more loving than my family was, why he'd want to go away when people who loved him were right here; and it hurt my feelings tremendously, because I really wanted to love him. My whole life I was looking for someone I could love because my parents never let me love them. It was very hard. But he would have a really great time, really enjoy something tremendously, and then he'd go into this despair.

After he divorced me, there was a short time when he wanted to go back to the way things were before we got married, and I withdrew; again, he pursued me, because that's how things always were. There was this big 180-degree flip, and after he divorced me he went back and was again so charismatic and had so much energy, and he brought presents. The day we got married, he didn't get wedding rings. He had two responsibilities, the wedding rings and where we were going to live. He didn't bring the wedding rings. We didn't have wedding rings on our wedding day. His sister went out and picked up something that morning that we used. I begged him for well over a year for a wedding ring and finally, just out of not wanting to hear me, got one. It was as if there was no sexual interest the whole time we were married; this persisted until he divorced me. I didn't know any better, because that's how I grew up in my own family. It was a very sad and tragic situation. We got divorced, and all of a sudden I was again being pursued, and he brought presents and had all of this energy again, but I wasn't going to go back. Once I was out of the situation, I got myself into analysis, I got help, started doing better, and I realized I felt better alone than in this relationship, and I didn't go back; especially because I saw this same ending coming. I saw that he was the same way that he was before he got married and saw what it led to, and I wasn't going back. So then we really didn't have a lot of contact because I realized that he wanted to resume the relationship, and my answer was no. So I needed to be firm about that. We just spoke intermittently, and this was probably 5 years ago. I know that soon thereafter he met his girlfriend. And he did the same thing with her. He never married her, but, and you'll probably hear this from her firsthand, things would be very good between them. They had a better relationship. I get real sensitive, and when he used to go into these 5- or 6-day retreats, it would really set me off. I didn't handle it well. It reminded me too much of my family situation when I was growing up; and, anyway, his girlfriend may not have this same vulnerability, and she is much more stable even. Anyway, things would be really good between them, and then he would break up with her. I think there were seven or eight backs and forths. At one point they were getting ready to elope, and he called and broke up with her. And it's the same pattern. The day we got married was the day when he reached his success, his goal; then he descended into despair because the pain was still there. I don't know the girlfriend very well, but I've met with her half a dozen times since Arthur's death. She is a lovely girl, I really like her.

ESS: *Are you sufficiently divorced from him to be happy in your life?*

EX-WIFE: Yes, I'm sure I am.

ESS: *What do you hope to be doing ten years from now?*

EX-WIFE: Living every day well, I hope. My biggest goal in life is to free myself from the misery I grew up in. I don't mean my own—I mean my father and my mother and Arthur, I'm starting to appreciate, are just such sick people with such misery inside. And I don't think I saw it and I didn't understand it; I learned my parents' way of seeing in the world, but I didn't know anything else. Then, when I moved in with Arthur, it didn't occur to me how bad it was and how ill he was. And now my biggest goal in life is to appreciate the beauty and the goodness in the world every single day and to live my life to the best I can and the most I can, without the things I am afraid of, the things that hurt. I'm just learning to really understand and appreciate the tragedy of my childhood and the tragedy of my marriage to Arthur, and I have to say, it feels really good to be in touch with it. And I think that's the thing about my parents, and Arthur as well. Both of my parents and Arthur would admit that they have pain. Arthur was always running to find something to fix it, and he never really looked into it and grappled with it. And the same with my parents. My parents had terrible things happen to them, and there is so much tragedy between them, they run from it. They deny it. My mother will look at me and say that she had a happy childhood. And I know she didn't because I know how she treats me and how she treated me when I was a child. And I know my father as well, I know that there is something so deeply saddening.

ESS: *If you were giving Arthur a psychiatric categorization, where would you put him?*

EX-WIFE: I don't know the answer to that, but I can tell you how I would summarize him. I'm not familiar enough with the *DSM* diagnoses, but I can tell you that he was extremely harsh toward himself and others, very judgmental. He believed in character, which I believe in, too, but. . . .

ESS: *What, the ability to rise above adversity and tough it out?*

EX-WIFE: Yes, and he was really a stickler about honesty. It was to such an extent that it was well beyond the normal.

ESS: *That he couldn't meet his own standards?*

EX-WIFE: Nobody could meet his standards. Which is why I think he hated himself so much for having asked me to talk to the dean, because he felt like he had cheated. It had nothing to do with his admission; anyone with logic would know. Inside he felt like a phony or fraud about himself. With all my intuition, that's what I would come up with. I don't tell a lot of people about my analysis or where I come from or about my experiences growing up. You know, I'm fortunate. I thank my analyst. I think it's just about the best thing I've ever done. But I do think about it sometimes, and I do realize that I've lived quite a bit.

ESS: *What could have been done for Arthur? Could his life have been saved?*

EX-WIFE: If someone could have helped him with that pain, yes, I think so.

ESS: *For example, do you think that your psychoanalyst could have saved him?*

EX-WIFE: I'd like to hope so. Yes, I would like to hope so. I think that if someone had focused on what it was that was hurting him so. Where do you hurt, and let's talk about it. Arthur would have resisted that because, like I said, he was always running from it. He was always looking outside. His running from that pain and not understanding it had to have been worse than if he could have actually seen it. But maybe it could have been done.

INTERVIEW WITH
THE GIRLFRIEND

ESS: *Please tell me who you are.*

GRL: Who am I? I'm Arthur's ex-girlfriend.

ESS: *Say a few words about yourself.*

GRL: I am 30 years old. I'm an office administrator for an engineering firm, and I have a wonderful family who live locally. I went on to college in this state, and after graduation with a psychology major I worked with disturbed adults for a couple of years. It was a lot of responsibility, and I was only 21 years old, so—I don't know how that happened. What broke my heart was that I became immune to it. I was thinking of case evaluations: When new clients would come to the clinic, I would do their intakes, and I remember the first few times I did it, it was hard; but after six months it became so routine, and that's one thing that I always look back on my life that it became routine, and these people were pouring out their hearts and souls to me, telling me when they first began to hear voices or when they first started becoming depressed, and I would just write it down and not really hear what they had to say.

ESS: *Do you feel guilty about that?*

GRL: Of course, I do, absolutely. You know my brother is a doctor and I know he tells me that, and I remember Arthur, too, they would tell me these things, that you have to become immune because it'll break you up. My mom has had some problems.

ESS: *Do you like her?*

GRL: Do I like her? I love her. I think she is a blessing. She is working at a school; she reads to kids and to elderly people at a convalescent home; I mean, she is the kind of person—when you're having a bad day or you're not happy with something, you look at her, and you say, Wow.

ESS: *Say something about your childhood.*

GRL: I had the most amazing childhood. My mother was a stay-at-home mom, and I just had an amazing childhood. My parents, my father is amazing, just very warm and loving. I had the classic nuclear family. When I'd come home—my father chose to have the kind of life where he didn't work really hard; I mean, he worked hard, he is an engineer, but he decided he would end his day at five o'clock so he'd come home and be with his family. And because of that his company didn't grow, it was just him as a sole practitioner, and he's done very well for himself for having a family; we ate dinner together every single night. My dad would take us out on weekends as a family, and my dad is just a very warm, loving, giving person.

ESS: *And how does Arthur fit into this?*

GRL: He was, the label is in the same category as my mother and my brother, that he was diagnosed with depression. He was a depressed individual. That's the label I would give him.

ESS: *Do you think it was bipolar disorder?*

GRL: Do I think that he had it? Well, I remember that he and I talked about it. I thought that it was a possibility, but I saw the very high manic part of it and I saw the very low, depressed part of it in other people. Arthur didn't have that high manic part, in my opinion, and again, that's just, because I worked with it firsthand with a lot of other people who were bipolar. But with Arthur, I didn't see the mania part; maybe the mania took part in a different form that I didn't recognize. I didn't see it with him the same way as I saw it in others. And being a psychology major, I studied that, too, and I know what some of those symptoms are, and Arthur didn't have them.

ESS: *What were your years with Arthur? When did you meet him?*

GRL: I met him 4 years ago this month.

ESS: *Was his marriage over by then?*

GRL: Yes.

ESS: *Have you met his ex-wife?*

GRL: Yes, but she was out of his life by then.

ESS: *You loved each other.*

GRL: Yes, very much.

ESS: *What was it about him that was lovable?*

GRL: He was really a good person with a really big heart. He was very caring and had a really big heart. He was very funny and smart, and he and I were very similar, like just being with him felt right and comfortable. We could talk about anything.

ESS: *You liked him.*

GRL: I liked him, yes; besides being in love with him, I really liked him.

ESS: *Did you break up with him?*

GRL: Oh, several times.

ESS: *What were those breakups about?*

GRL: Well, we were together for a year, and during that year I thought that everything was perfect, and it really was perfect up until I went to Spain. His family invited me to come with them. So I went to Spain. He had left, I think, two weeks before all of us, and we went to meet him; and I just remember going to see him and that he didn't seem overjoyed. You know, I was so on the tips of my toes, and I jumped and hugged him, and I just felt something weird. I just remember that it was in Spain. And when we came back, he told me that he just wasn't happy any more, that he just wasn't happy.

ESS: *Not happy with you, with life, with what?*

GRL: It's funny because at the time I thought it was with the relation-ship, but later he told me that it wasn't me at all; it was life, he just wasn't feeling good. He and I broke up probably three or four times; and it was always him coming back to me, and I'd accept him back.

ESS: *What would he say?*

GRL: When he'd come back? Exactly what I just said, that it wasn't me. He realized that it wasn't me that made him unhappy; he was just not a happy person, and he wasn't happy with life, and he thought our breaking up and him dating other people might make him happy; and when he did, he realized it wasn't that at all; and that I really did make him feel good when we were together. I think he realized that we had a really good thing going, a really good relationship, and him being down had nothing to do with our relationship.

ESS: *You think this was he speaking or his pathology speaking?*

GRL: I think it was a combination of both. I think Arthur was an incred-ibly smart person, and that was the problem with his illness. Some-body who doesn't understand the mind and the psychology of the mind won't understand they're sick. He was the kind of person who understood what happiness was but wasn't able to find it within himself, and because he couldn't find it, it made him even more depressed.

ESS: *What's the "it"?*

GRL: I don't even know if he couldn't find the happiness or if he couldn't make the sadness go away. I know he had times of joy. He told me when we first met that the first few months we were together he really was happy, he was truly happy; he told me that. And Arthur and I used to talk about this all the time, his depression and how he felt; and that was one wonderful thing about our relationship—he knew that I understood him because I had already lived it. And so he was able to be so open with me because he knew I understood, and I knew how to take care of him. I don't know if that makes any sense, but I think that's why our relationship was so deep, because of that.

ESS: *How did you take care of him?*

GRL: I think I took care of him, I think part of it was just letting him know that I understood how he felt; and I let him feel down when he wanted to feel down, and I let him know that I was there to take care of him. And when you feel a certain way and you know you're not supposed to feel that way—like, he knew that he was sick. And when you know that, and you know there is someone else there that loves you, that understands that exact thing that you're going through, that's an amazing feeling. It did not make him feel entirely good, but it made him feel truly loved. And he can't feel joy, but maybe he can feel it some, I don't know—I'm just throwing that out there. He knew that I understood and I do, to this day I still understand. I don't understand other things, but it's just something that I do.

ESS: *You were his friend, his lover, his psychiatric nurse.*

GRL: I didn't analyze, I never did that, but I did take care of him; and that's almost in my nature, too. When you really love somebody, you do all those things.

ESS: *And then what happened?*

GRL: The first time we broke up, for me it was most devastating, and I'll never forget it. I had had boyfriends before, but this was the first time I was fully in love, and I cried for two weeks. It was the weirdest thing. This sounds so terrible, but I cried, I was in more pain then than when he actually passed away. I know it sounds terrible to say that, but even now I feel that way.

ESS: *Like the death of part of you.*

GRL: It was awful. But soon it started to get better and then, of course, he called me and we got back together.

ESS: *That happened more than once?*

GRL: Yes. The first time he called me, I went over to his house, and he told me we were just going to talk, and, of course, he told me that he wanted me back; and he said to me that those last two weeks were the worst two weeks of his life, too, and so we got back together. And we were together probably for another two or three months. Things would be great the first month, and then it started to do the same thing again, and I think we broke up again and, truthfully, at that point it was hard, it was really hard for me, but it was nothing like those first two weeks. I don't know why, but it was just a little bit easier. Maybe because I knew something more. And then we got back together another couple of times, and then at some point I just couldn't take it anymore, and I said, "enough," and then, finally, of course, when I said, "I can't do this anymore," that's when he kept calling me.

ESS: *What stage were you in when he died? A state of separation between you two?*

GRL: Yes, we were definitely separated, but we were in contact. Arthur called me Friday night, and my then boyfriend was actually at my house when Arthur called me, I think it was like one or two o'clock in the morning. He called me, and he had told me many times that he was going to kill himself. I mean, this was something that was not the first time I heard that. And that night he called me again and said, "You know, I can't take it anymore. If you don't get back together with me—if I'm not with you—I'm going to kill myself." And he said it in so many words; and I was worried. We talked for about an hour and—jumping back—there were other times when he had done this. I remember one time he had done this, and I called his sister and told her that he was threatening to kill himself. This particular night he did it, and—I know this sounds terrible—I took it seriously, I did, but I took it as seriously as I did the other 20 times. So we talked, and when I hung up he had promised me he wasn't going to kill himself. The next morning, I flew out of town, and I called him from the airport to say, "How are you doing," just to check up on him and make sure he was doing okay. Sure enough, he was in a great mood; he was going out with his pal and everything was fine, and he sounded like his normal self. So I felt better, and that was it. I thought, okay, whatever he told me last night was just a bad time. So I felt good, and I visited my friend, returned, and on Monday—and I was going to call him on Monday and just didn't get a chance to call—and then on the way out his sister called me on Monday night and told me.

ESS: *What were your first reactions?*

GRL: Oh, I'll never forget. My knees just buckled, and I collapsed to the ground, screaming. I just said "No, No, No" over and over again, and, to be honest, when she called me, I knew before she said it, and I always knew. One of the reasons, toward the end, I didn't want to get back together with him and I didn't want to marry him was that I knew in the back of my mind that someday he would kill himself; and I knew that, I did know that.

ESS: *You knew that you'd have a roller coaster ride?*

GRL: I knew that I would have that. But my fear was that we would get married, have children, and then he'd kill himself, and I would be all alone. I had a dream about Arthur recently, and I would think about him every single day. But I don't think it will stop, I hope it doesn't. I'll never stop thinking about Arthur, never. He was a good man.

ESS: *The question has to be asked: What might or could have been done to have saved him?*

GRL: I think about that all the time. I should have told his mom, been stronger and said that he is going to kill himself, he really is.

ESS: *What would she then be obligated to do?*

GRL: When I was driving over here, I thought about that—what could I have done?

ESS: *What could have been done by anybody?*

GRL: Nothing, nothing. Let me tell you why. I shouldn't say "nothing." Arthur was such a smart person. He used to say to me—because I used to tell him, "You need to go to the hospital," or "I'm going to send you to a hospital"—and he used to always say: "I'm too smart for that. You have me admitted to a hospital, and I'm going to know exactly how to act, exactly what I'm supposed to do, and they'll release me, and meanwhile you'll have ruined my life because I'll lose everything in my life. I will have really lost face with my friends and my family, and I'll probably kill myself." And he would look me straight in the eye and tell me that. He had to have wanted to be helped. And the sad thing is, I know he wanted to be helped so badly.

ESS: *He was in pain, in great pain. What was the nature of that pain?*

GRL: He would say to me, he would want me to understand what this pain felt like. And he would say it felt like lying on a bed of needles, that the pain was so intense, it went into every bit of his body, and that's exactly what he would say, that it felt like lying on a bed of needles.

ESS: *It doesn't quite answer the question that I have on my mind. I'm not sure exactly how to ask it, but I'll ask it this way: What was the nature of his mental pain? Being on a bed of needles is physical torture. What was the nature of his mental pain?*

GRL: It's hard for me to answer that question because—it's to say he was very sad or depressed, or couldn't feel any joy, or—that doesn't do it justice. That's like a slap in the face.

ESS: *There's a word for that: anhedonia.*

GRL: Yes, he used to talk about that.

ESS: *But that simply says that one is depressed and sad. I'm searching for what's behind that. What was he depressed and sad about? That he was ugly? That he was stupid? That he was unsuccessful?*

GRL: Yes, and I'm surprised that no one else has said this to you, but he used to say that he used to do really badly in school.

ESS: *I'm looking for paradigms. I'm looking for little hints of the larger picture.*

GRL: I'll tell you something that he once said to me that relates to that. He once said that when he first would date a woman, the thing that gave him the biggest amount of joy was when he would first sleep with her; he said that actually made him really happy. And then, afterwards, it was not so good.

ESS: *What, the conquest?*

GRL: Maybe. I don't know. But he used to tell me that that actually did make him happy, and I always thought that was a little odd, but he did tell me that before. I don't know if that helps you at all.

ESS: *Well, it's difficult to live a life where your joys come from first times. Because there are a lot of activities which are repetitive and sustained, and there is a first time, and then you're disappointed when it's the second and the third time.*

GRL: And that makes sense with our relationship. Maybe after almost a year, there was no more first time, and he wasn't happy any more.

ESS: *Tell me some things about Arthur's psychotherapist. I have not met him yet.*

GRL: I've never met him, either. If Arthur would stay Friday night, on Saturday he'd get up and actually go to his appointment with him. I never met him. I think he's called me once to see where Arthur was when he was running late, but I didn't speak to him. I just know that, from hearing other people speak of him, that he has been seeing him for years and years, and it seems to me that it was more like two old friends talking than the doctor helping him. It just seemed like they were just too used to each other, and they would just sit and talk for an hour.

ESS: *What did Arthur say about him? Did he like him?*

GRL: Yes. He did like him, but he didn't think that he was helping him so much.

ESS: *Did he ever say: "My psychotherapist is the one who can save my life?" Or did he ever say: "My psychotherapist can't save my life?"*

GRL: No, he didn't say that, either. I don't know if this is from listening to people talk this past year and a half, but I think this doctor was the one Arthur started going to after he attempted it the first time as an adolescent. I don't recall that, it's not strong in my mind. I do recall that Arthur never said, "He can save my life."

ESS: *You don't have animosity toward Arthur's psychotherapist?*

GRL: No, not a bit.

ESS: *Have you seen Arthur's suicide note? What were your reactions to the note?*

GRL: At the time, just this broken-hearted feeling. I think I was more concerned with his death than anybody.

ESS: *Did you feel indicted or accused in any way?*

GRL: No, he didn't make anyone feel that way.

ESS: *Do you feel you were the love of his life?*

GRL: I think I was one love of his life. I think his wife was a love of his life, too. I think the same situation that happened with me happened with her, as well. I think they really loved each other a lot, but I knew that someday this was going to happen; even though I still wanted to marry him. I mean, he was the love of my life, and I know that he loved me so much, too. He was definitely the love of my life, and that's it. But I don't want you to think that my love for my husband is different. I think Arthur was born with his illness. I definitely feel that way. This feeling of not being able to feel, this depression that he felt was an illness that he was born with. And I'm a strong believer in that, just as you have a physical illness such as cancer, you have psychological illness that can kill you, and that's what killed him. It was like having a cancer for all the years of his life, and it finally took over his body. He was born with it. I'll always believe that. It's different when you get depressed for other reasons, but this wasn't that kind of depression. Some people don't understand mental illness. A lot of people don't, and I feel like I do. That's why I think he was born with it. He has wonderful parents. His mom is a wonderful person. Sure, she got on his nerves; she got on my nerves, too, but I love her, and she has so much love inside her. And his dad, he is a good person, too. His parents were divorced, but plenty of people have divorced parents.

ESS: *You don't think the acrimony of that divorce seared Arthur in a special way?*

GRL: I do think it was tough on him. But look at his brother and sisters. If he were an only child, you could look at that more closely, but he was not. His mom told me he had problems when he was a little kid, too, even before the divorce. And I know, it's so hard, I can't tell that to his mom or his dad or anyone, but I feel—and it's hard to express it to you even—but I feel like I do understand. I feel like I understand why he did it, and I wished to God that I could have helped him; I tried, I really did. But I feel like I understand why he did it, I feel like I understand his pain. The night was his enemy; because when he was alone at home, and the sun would go down, he would sit on his couch and he would just sink down. But we would go out on the weekends and during the week. I mean, we had fun. I wouldn't have spent all that time with him had he been in this depression 24–7. He was a fun loving, goodhearted, and a very loving person, very smart. One time we went miniature golfing after we had broken up several times, and I was just with him because I knew he needed to get out of the house. We went miniature golfing and played all these games, and we won all these tickets to win prizes with, and he found such great joy passing them out to all the kids. I wanted to buy something stupid, and he said, "No, let's pass them out to all the kids." And he went around to all the kids, asking, "Do you want some tickets, do you want some?" I mean he loved doing that, that's the kind of man he was. He was a really good man. We gave and we took from each other. When you write about him, I just want you to know that he was all those other wonderful things.

INTERVIEW WITH
THE PSYCHOTHERAPIST

ESS: *Please tell me how you knew Arthur.*

PSY: Basically, I knew him at three different phases of his life. I originally met him when he was a young boy and the parents brought
him in to me because he was having a lot of difficulties. He was an
angry, unhappy, difficult child, and I saw him. He might have been
around 8 or so. He was one of the angriest children that I have seen
in over 30 years of practice. In the beginning, he was physically
almost unmanageable at times. I would have to hold him and
restrain him. He once punched me in the groin so hard he doubled
me over. He tried to pull my bookcases down. He ran off one time,
and I had to carry him back for several blocks. In some respects, he
was one of the most difficult children I have ever seen. My understanding at the time was that much of this was a reaction to his parents' relatively contentious divorce. There was no love lost between
the parents. Treatment went well. He improved dramatically, and
we terminated treatment ultimately because things were going well,
and he was in a good place and things were going well in school.

ESS: *Tell me about treatment. What was that like?*

PSY: My background may have become more eclectic over the years, but
it was very psychodynamically oriented. I was trained at a psychoanalytic child study center with an analytic understanding and
approach to things. We usually used the vehicle of play. You let the
child choose what they wanted to do and talk about, and ultimately
where they are drawn to and how they express themselves is a reflection of their issues, and often by direct interpretation or through the
vehicle of play the therapist will respond to what those issues are

and help them work it through. My understanding is, what makes this approach effective is a combination of the cathartic aspect of working through the issues experientially in the sessions, as well as the insights that are gleaned and unconscious material that is brought to the forefront. I had all kinds of objects in the office: games, dart guns, family puppets. Like I said, we terminated treatment because, thankfully, he was no longer being physical with me, and things were much better on the home front and in school. I don't remember exactly how some of this got played out on the home front.

ESS: *But he was an angry child?*

PSY: Very.

ESS: *What did he say? At whom was he angry?*

PSY: Again, my understanding was that the target of the anger was the parents, the siblings in some respects. Some of that I'll get into when I talk about the three phases of my treatment with him. Some of what I was able to then speak with him about when he was older and able to communicate more articulately also shed light on the earlier phase of treatment. But I do recall my understanding of it was, the dynamics that were getting played out were related to what I described to you. Then we terminated treatment because things went well at home and in school. I didn't hear from the family for quite a few years. Then, one night, I got a phone call in the middle of the night when he was 15 or so, that he had made a suicide attempt by overdose. I had gotten a phone call that he was at the hospital, they were pumping his stomach, he had overdosed on pills. At that point I began meeting with him again. The treatment obviously was no longer using play as the vehicle. We talked about what he was feeling and thinking, and it was during the course of that second phase of his treatment that he was able to talk about his insecurities. I'm not completely clear which of those sometimes came out during the second phase of the treatment or when he called me later as an adult; but he was very insecure at that point; he didn't have a lot of confidence in himself, was concerned about his relationships and that the other kids did not think highly of him.

ESS: *Are you saying those feelings were implicated in his suicide attempt at that time?*

PSY: There was not one particular thing that broke the camel's back, so to speak. My sense of it is, it was more just sort of the overwhelming sense of unhappiness with his life and himself. It was at this point that he was able to begin to talk more articulately about things, like feeling that the father really cared much more about the older brother than he did about him. The older brother was, at least at that time, thought to be brighter. He was at a private high school, and he was on the basketball team, and I think that for Arthur the older brother, at that time, represented to him what he wished he were and felt he could not be; and he definitely felt that the father cared more about the older brother than he did about him. I think this even translated into the symbolism of money that was spent on him, and the feeling that the father didn't take care of him financially as well as he could have. That was a very significant theme in the third phase of treatment, but I think we saw the beginnings of it in the second phase; the father was spending more money on his second wife, and Arthur felt that was sort of symbolic of his not caring enough for him.

He always spoke of the discomfort that he felt with his mother. After he committed suicide, she lamented the fact that she knew she never really had the closeness with him that she wished she could have had. And he was never really able to concisely articulate what it was about his mother that he couldn't connect with; but it was clear that there was a real discomfort with her. He was uncomfortable in her presence; and what was most puzzling about this, as even he and I talked about it, it was not like she ever did anything negative to him, like he perceived the father as being withholding and not giving enough. Mother really tried very hard to connect with him, and it made it all the more puzzling, even to Arthur, why it didn't sit well with him. And the best that I've been able to make out of this is that I always experienced mother as someone who really cared about Arthur and was basically a good, decent person; but there was a quality about her that was a little hard to articulate, but it had something to do with the idea that she seemed very needy, and she seemed like somebody who, when caught up in her own needs, could sort of suck you dry in terms of like what she was needy for. I don't know how else to explain it.

ESS: *Do you think he was afraid of that quality in her?*

PSY: Again, you could make a good theoretical case for the fact that it was fear, but he never described it as fear. The closest that he was able to get to talking about it was that she made him feel uncomfortable. He knew he could depend upon her. She was the one he would come to; that's why I say it was really confusing for him. It was confusing for me.

ESS: *That's a very subtle thing.*

PSY: Yes. It was something that, as I say, in his adolescent and adult treatment we talked about quite tangibly. He was never really able to definitively articulate what this quality was, but it was there from the time he was very young, and it never went away. You just sort of got the feeling that somehow, in the very early phase of life, in the bonding between the two of them, something went awry; and I was never really able to understand what it was, but it was early, and it never went away.

ESS: *That there was some idiosyncratic pathological character to it?*

PSY: As I say, it's confusing, and I've always wished I could have understood it better. I never really felt that I had a clear sense of it, in great part because Arthur never had a clear sense of it. It's something that we talked about a lot during his second and third treatment phase.

ESS: *Did you discuss this case with anyone at that time?*

PSY: I don't remember to whom I talked about it, but I didn't go in for supervision.

ESS: *What was your sense, when this adolescent suicide attempt occurred, about the prognosis of this case?*

PSY: Initially, obviously, I was uncertain; but, again, over the course of time we made significant headway. He felt better about himself, he felt better about his life, he was developing good peer relationships, he began to take pride in his own intellect. We made a lot of headway in terms of his self-esteem, and he began to believe that, even though he may not have been, in his mind, as bright as his brother, that he was still somebody who was intelligent and had a lot to offer. Again, it had a very positive evolution.

ESS: *How often did you see him?*

PSY: It was at least once a week, but I saw him twice a week in the early phases.

ESS: *Do you feel that he liked you?*

PSY: I'm sure he liked me.

ESS: *Apparently he did.*

PSY: I'm sure he liked me, and I feel that I can say that he continued to come to see me, and what makes me feel secure that he really felt comfortable with me was that, as an adult, when he came back, he chose me; he could have gone to anyone else. We really had very good rapport.

ESS: *Did you like him?*

PSY: Yes, I did. It was a little bit harder to like him when he was punching me in the groin, but, ultimately, he was a likeable person, and I enjoyed my sessions with him. I remember, in the second phase of his treatment, that the nature of our schedule was such that it worked out best for him to see me at the end of the day; but then he was going to have trouble getting over to his after-school appointment. I used to drive him to that appointment on the way home because it was in the direction of where I lived. So we had what I would call a very comfortable relationship together, and I had trust in him.

Things were very good, and I didn't hear from him for a number of years after that. Then, the third phase of our work together was when he called me as an adult, when he was in medical school. At this point, when he called me, he was quite depressed initially. The issues, again, interestingly enough, were similar in some respects, as you might anticipate, despite the fact that he was clearly a very bright kid. He had gotten accepted to medical school because he wanted to be a physician like his father. Part of what caused him to start getting back into that insecure, second-guessing, sort of, approach to things for himself was that he questioned whether he had really gotten into medical school on his own, or if it was that his wife was accepted as well, and so they just sort of brought him along with her. He was very hard on himself, was very concerned that he was not going to be adequate to be a doctor or a lawyer. He was afraid that he wouldn't be able to make good choices for people. Despite the fact that he had so much success in various ways, it didn't really register as deeply as one would hope for in terms of how he felt about himself. A major piece of our work together in that period of time focused on what that was all about for him, and how irrational and unrealistic some of his perspectives were. It was as if, if he wasn't the best, then he was nothing at all; the best or nothing. And, again, it was something we very tangibly worked on together, and, again, that part of it improved significantly, and he began to feel more adequate in that respect. That was the kind of pressure he put on himself.

Now, some of what this was all about—and it tied in with depression, but it may have tied in, obviously, with other things as well—he had a lot of difficulty getting himself to study, and he would procrastinate tremendously. So, often his perception was that he didn't do as well as he could have, because he hadn't put in the time and the energy that was necessary to pull it off. And yet, again, as I had pointed out to him, that was really a testimony as to how bright [he was] and what his potential really was that he was able to do as well as he did without putting in a full effort, and I think he started to eventually get that.

He struggled a lot with the feeling that he really didn't have the kind of feelings for his wife that he wished he had. There was a lot of guilt that we had to work through in that regard. He sort of felt he had married her for the wrong reasons; that, in his insecurities, he too quickly made something happen just so he would be with somebody, but that she really wasn't quite the right person for him. But, again, he perceived her as a good person, that he didn't want to hurt her but clearly was not happy with her. I think that the focus of his discontent was more that he felt he didn't find her physically as attractive as he wished she had been; and, again, that was similar to the other girl that he wound up with. Maybe that will help capture the flavor, because it is applicable to both the wife and the girlfriend. I think, in the context of the insecurities that he struggled with, he was the kind of person who fantasized about having a certain kind of woman he would really find attractive but [he] never thought he was good enough to have that kind of woman, so he settled for women that weren't what he really wanted; but then he was always disappointed because he knew he settled. And they were always good people, he never questioned them in terms of being good decent human beings, but just on a chemistry level. Physically, the women he wound up getting were not as high up as what he really wished, and then he didn't feel the kind of excitement with them that he wanted to feel. It never was anything that ultimately he could put his finger on in terms of what that sort of deeper part of things might have been all about; the part that was most tangible was, his insecurities were such that he didn't give himself a chance to really go for the kind of woman he thought could really make him happy.

ESS: *That he wasn't good enough to merit the kind of person he really wanted. And that he never would be?*

PSY: I think that when he stopped treatment the third time, it was my sense that he felt, "You know what, I actually made it out of two professional schools; lots of women like doctors and lawyers and if for no other reason than that they make a lot of money." My sense of it was, he was going out into the world feeling that maybe now he had a better chance than he did before. He didn't stop treatment at that point with a sense of pessimism, on that I am clear.

ESS: *Please say something about the stopping of treatment.*

PSY: This sort of happened casually. A lot of it he attributed to a combination of his schedule having become much more demanding and that he was feeling better, there wasn't as much a sense of urgency to come in as before. I had explored with him whether there was some reticence to coming in at that point, but that was nothing he ever acknowledged.

ESS: *Was he suicidal when he stopped treatment?*

PSY: At the point when he stopped treatment, I didn't think that he was. He had suicidal ideation during the course of that period of time. One of the things that I haven't mentioned yet: He was initially very resistant to taking medication; he saw it as a failure, yet another sign of inadequacy on his part, and so we had to do a lot of work to get him to agree to the medication. Ultimately, he did. My recollection is that the first psychiatrist I sent him to he didn't quite hit it off with; he wound up with somebody else. What stands out in my mind is that he felt it helped him dramatically but that he had to be sure to take it on time; otherwise, he would get headaches. He felt it made a significant difference.

One of the things that he and I had talked about was, often, life didn't feel very appealing and enjoyable to him when he was feeling very depressed, obviously; but that also some of it was sort of similar, in the vein of not giving himself the chance to go after that "A" girl that he was always hoping for. He didn't really give himself a chance to do the things that did bring him a lot of pleasure; and so one of the things that we started working on was what was getting in the way of that and what could we do to help him to begin to access things that he did get some enjoyment out of. And so, one of the things that ultimately he gave himself a chance to do and enjoyed was to join a Scrabble club, and he went to play Scrabble several times a week, and he seemed to derive satisfaction and enjoyment out of that. He was very bright and very good at it. Interestingly enough, in that regard—and I saw that as a sign of a facet of the improvement that he had made—that he realized he wasn't the best Scrabble player. I mean, these were obviously the primo Scrabble players in the city, but he was okay with that, he didn't have to be the very best. He was able to still enjoy it and felt that he could hold his own, and he did it.

During this period of time he ultimately did divorce his wife, and we worked through that. They were already separated, but what I remember for sure is we worked through his guilt about that. And then there was this other woman who came into his life. Again, she was a very nice girl and he liked her, but he never felt that passion for her that he wished he could have felt for a woman. A lot of that, again, had to do with the feeling on his part that he was settling. But not settling in the sense they weren't good people, but settling just in the sense there wasn't the kind of chemistry there that he fantasized. It had eluded him to the point where we stopped treatment, but at that point he had made so much headway in so many other ways that I had the feeling that he might ultimately give himself a chance. One of the reasons I did feel so encouraged at that time that life could have gone well for him at that point—he felt good about having completed his education as both a physician and an attorney; he did feel that had given him a certain amount of stature. He felt that he would be a good enough professional when he actually started working. I remember we talked about the fact, about making good decisions, and he did feel that he could help people. So there seemed clearly to be a better sense of self that he had come to. As I said, while there was no way for me to be sure at that point, I did have the feeling that he might ultimately give himself a chance to go for the kind of relationship that he was looking for.

ESS: *That was how many months or years before his death?*

PSY: I stopped seeing him approximately 2½ years before he killed himself.

ESS: *Were there any contacts between you two during that time?*

PSY: I had called him at one point to see how he was doing. My recollection is that he felt good, things were going well, and he sent me a nice note at one point, saying how much he enjoyed our meetings together and how much I had helped him.

ESS: *Were you totally surprised when he killed himself?*

PSY: When you say total—I guess once somebody has tried it, you realize there is always the possibility that it may happen again, but I was very surprised. I don't think I've mentioned this, but during the third phase of treatment, it was clear at that point how much physiology was driving the depression.

ESS: *Say more about that.*

PSY: I felt pretty secure at that point that it wasn't just a psychologically based response, and that's why I wanted to be sure that he was on medication.

ESS: *How do you conceptualize the biology of this?*

PSY: In retrospect, hindsight being twenty-twenty as they say, I was pretty suspicious that there was physiology, biology, going through this, all through the course of time. What made me, I think, more dubious of that during the earlier phases of my work with him was how much success we had without using medication. It was my feeling that if it had really been, in those periods of time, primarily or in great part biology driven, as you said, I would not have anticipated that we could achieve as much dramatic improvement as we had.

ESS: *What? A kind of endogenous depression?*

PSY: As I look back on it now, I'd be pretty suspicious of that at this point, okay?

ESS: *And how do you conceptualize this?*

PSY: My guess would be that he was born with it and that the difficulties in the environment then exacerbated what was a vulnerability in this regard.

ESS: *Do you see him as star-crossed, that is, there was a kind of inevitability of this outcome in this case?*

PSY: No, that was not how I explain it, no; and the reason that I felt, I can say that clearly just now, was that he responded well to the medication. I mean it wasn't a panacea, it wasn't like everything went away, but it was a significant improvement, at least during the time I knew him; and he was making healthier choices for himself and feeling better about those choices. Especially after he had become a physician, he seemed to feel that he had opportunities and potential that I don't think he saw for himself before that, and I think he felt that he had accomplished something, and he wanted to help people, and he seemed to feel that he was achieving that. For example, he wasn't the kind of person who became a doctor or lawyer to make a lot of money; he seemed really sincere in wanting to help people, and when last I spoke to him, he seemed to be feeling good about the fact that he thought he was, in fact, able to do that. That was a couple of years before his death.

ESS: *We ought to, please, address the perplexing theoretical question of how might he have been saved. What could have saved him?*

PSY: Obviously, that is the question that I have been struggling with since his death. And, quite honestly, when you called me, one of the things I was curious whether you could give me any insight on it. As I reviewed what he and I had done together, I couldn't think of anything—this sounds like a self-serving statement—that I could have done something differently. Like I say, he seemed in a better place, his life seemed to be going much better.

ESS: *Would it have helped if he had been in psychotherapy at that time?*

PSY: I would hope so, but for some reason at that point he didn't. Have you seen the letter that he wrote, the long suicide note?

ESS: *Yes, I have a copy.*

PSY: He made it clear in that what had evolved ultimately was a sense of feeling that the good times never stayed long enough; the gist of it was that it always came back again to the darkness, and that he no longer had the hope that he could stay consistently okay.

ESS: *Yes, that notion haunted him.*

PSY: But that was not the sense of who he was when I saw him last. That's part of what made it so terribly sad to see that he ultimately had concluded that, because, as I say, if you go back to, as I say, as fate would have it, these three different phases of his life that I knew him, we were always able to get things to a much better place for him.

ESS: *Did you puzzle as to why he didn't reach out for you?*

PSY: Yes, I did, and I don't know. One of the things I wondered about was whether the biology had become so overpowering at that point that he couldn't even see. For him, to call me the third time required still enough belief and hope that things would get better that he let me in the door, so to speak; and I can only assume by the time of the suicide that, whatever I had been able to give him before, he no longer was able to remember or connect with or feel that it would be enough.

ESS: *Do you think that it would have helped if you had called him and told him he ought to come in to see you?*

PSY: I did, at one point, say that. I had made a phone call to him, but his contention at that point was that things were going sufficiently well and that it really wasn't necessary. I mean, I did reach out to him.

ESS: *You can't do more than that. The word* pain *is repeated throughout the suicide note. In the first paragraph, it's used several times, in the first short sentence: "I can't stand this pain, this pain is overwhelming, this pain is just too awful."*

PSY: The pain of hopelessness that he felt; the pain of not seeing the light at the end of the tunnel; the pain of there being nothing in life at that point that brought him any joy. When he gave me the chance to work with him, we always got to a better place; that's why I was so profoundly saddened that he didn't reach out to me again. It wasn't like we ever stopped treatment because I couldn't help him. Obviously, there are some cases where people stop because things are not getting any better. We always stopped because things had been significantly better, and that's what made this time around, where he didn't access me, all the more tragic.

ESS: *In a sense, you have implied the important role of biology.*

PSY: Yes, at this point, that's what I would say. Biology, then exacerbated by difficulties in life. Although, without the biology, I don't think those difficulties in life were powerful enough to lead someone to suicide. Yes. That's how I would look at it at this point, yes, that we are dealing with probably, assuming that he was genetically predisposed.

ESS: *Did you ever give him a* Diagnostic and Statistical Manual *diagnosis?*

PSY: Obviously, diagnostically, major depression at the end there. I didn't see him as psychotic.

ESS: *What role did his parents' contentious divorce play in his life? Do you think he would have been any different if there had been no divorce, no contention?*

PSY: That is what we would call the 64,000-dollar question. Barring something that happened to him that none of us are aware of, some other kind of trauma or molestation, which I have no reason at this point to believe, the reason that I keep coming back to the physiology of it is, we have a brother and sisters who have their issues, but neither of them were taken down by the family dynamics the way he was. So that's why what I said before seems to me the most parsimonious explanation at this point: that we have this biological, physiological vulnerability, and then the difficulties of the family played on that.

CONSULTATION BY
DAVID RUDD, PH.D.

David Rudd, who is in his 40s, is professor of psychology and director of train-
ing in clinical psychology at Baylor University. His doctoral degree is from the
University of Texas, and he held a postdoctoral fellowship in cognitive therapy
under Dr. Aaron T. Beck in Philadelphia. He has written more than seventy
publications on cognitive therapy and on treating suicidal behavior. He is cur-
rently president of the American Association of Suicidology.

Suicide is a loss of human potential, a loss of love and intimacy, a loss
of creativity and hope; in short, a loss of the preciousness that is life.
It is a loss that reaches far beyond the bounds of the individual. This is
clear from the interviews so elegantly conducted by Dr. Shneidman.
Rather than putting an end to emotional suffering, it has transformed
itself into something different, a new brand of suffering or psychache—
a legacy of pain and loss. After reading the interviews, one can have little doubt that suffering persists. We see this in the persistent questions of
the relatives and their efforts to explain the loss; it is even evident in the
suicide note, with its numerous apologies and reassurances.

Suicide is embedded in the social fabric of our lives. We are not isolated beings, existing separate and distinct from one another. Rather, we
are inextricably intertwined, to a depth and complexity that becomes
painfully apparent when there is a suicide. Suicide ripples into the
extended family system and into the larger community, immediately
and for generations to come. The loss leaves a painful legacy that lives
on in the persistent question, Why? It's a loss that is felt in the psyches of
those left behind, in some sense a new brand of psychache. Psychache is

"the hurt, anguish, soreness, aching, psychological pain in the psyche, the mind" (Shneidman, 1993, p. 51). What we see in the text and language of the interviews is psychache in a new form—that manifested by a suicide survivor. It is evident in every interview, in the questions asked and the explanations given.

I shall approach this case from a somewhat special perspective, one founded in cognitive theory but bolstered and influenced heavily by modern psychological theory, specifically Murray's notion of psychological needs (1938) and Shneidman's (1993) construct and theory of psychache. The theories are quite complementary, with an integration of them reflecting the richness, depth, and complexity of the human personality. Cognitive theory advances the idea of *modes*. A mode refers to the specific suborganizations within the personality organization that incorporate the cognitive (information processing), affective, behavioral, and motivational systems of the personality. The component parts of the mode are interactive and interdependent.

The original conceptualization of the mode has been expanded to account for a suicide-specific mode (Rudd, Joiner, & Rajab, 2000). Within the mode, a range of things can trigger a *suicidal cycle*. The defining feature of the suicidal mode, at least from a cognitive perspective, is the suicidal belief system, a construct that incorporates the individual's suicidal beliefs, those beliefs traditionally thought of as being dominated by hopelessness. In short, the suicidal belief system is a means of verbalizing the individual's psychache. How does the patient put his psychological pain and suffering into words? The suicidal belief system is how individual psychache is understood; it thus provides a tangible target for the therapist. What does the patient make of the inner, felt psychache? It is the patient's way of identifying what needs have been frustrated or thwarted. For each theme (discussed here) of the suicidal belief system, identifiable psychological needs have been frustrated. "Hopelessness" is too broad a concept to be useful in individual cases; it needs to be individually tailored to be effective in the clinical encounter.

It is perhaps easiest to understand suicide from a linear time perspective, moving from a triggering event (internal or external) to activation of the belief system, concomitant emotional and physiological response, and behavior that facilitates (or impedes) the patient's suicidality. In Arthur's case, the opening line of his note encapsulates his psychache and the core of his suicidal belief system: "All I do is suffer each and every day. Every moment is pain and numbness. How long can I do without pleasure?"

In a much more detailed manner than the construct of hopelessness, I propose four central themes to the suicidal belief system, all but one of which are seen in Arthur: (1) unlovability ("I don't deserve to live"); (2) helplessness ("I can't solve my problems"); (3) poor distress tolerance, or psychache ("I can't stand this pain any more"); and (4) perceived burdensomeness ("Everyone would be better off if I were dead"). In this case, the only theme not identified by Arthur in his suicide note or from interviews was *unlovability*. As an adult, he seemed to recognize his skills and inherent ability, although at a young age this was not necessarily the case. As a child and adolescent, all four themes were likely active in his suicidal belief system. What is clear from the interviews with his parents, brother, psychologist, and psychiatrist is the long-standing nature of his dysphoria and suffering. From a cognitive standpoint, this is the central problem. Over time, he came to believe that his suffering was intolerable (psychache and poor distress tolerance) and that it could not be changed or effectively treated (helplessness). Similarly, he had started to interpret the chronicity of his illness and problems as a burden to others (perceived burdensomeness). His death would not only relieve *his* suffering but also the suffering of others. In one of the most striking interviews, his psychiatrist indicates that he had bought into this belief system ("I vividly remember his first visit because my impression was, clearly, that some day he was going to commit suicide"). Even if carefully guarded against in the sessions, there are often subtle, covert, and implicit tie-ins with this sense of helplessness and hopelessness. The sense of helplessness is also evident in the interviews with the mother and father, as well as the brother. It is critical for the clinician to identify the suicidal belief system and directly target and monitor it in therapy. Failure to identify, target, and monitor the suicidal belief system runs the risk of reinforcing it.

The early developmental trajectory described in the interviews provides a fertile foundation for Arthur's suicidal belief system, across all four themes (unlovability, helplessness, poor distress tolerance or psychache, and perceived burdensomeness). Clearly, his temperament was hypersensitive. How did his parents interpret this? It is clear that they identified his problems early on and sought out care and treatment. In short, there was a problem; he was somehow deficient and didn't quite measure up to his brother. How did the patient interpret this? How did he make sense of it? From the information we have, it would appear that he came to the same conclusion as his parents, that he was somewhat deficient in some way. Early in his life he may well have identified himself as unlovable, something that never changed as his obvious successes (and evidence to the contrary) mounted. The foundation for his sense of helplessness is apparent in his history, in terms of the recurrent and persistent nature of his dysphoria and his emotional isolation and related anhedonia. He seems to have latched on to a biological explanation, acknowledging little individual control and influence on the course of his depression. As is evident in his suicide note, as the problems persist, his tolerance wanes, and his sense of being a burden grows. As I read his suicide note and the interviews, I found myself wondering to what degree he understood his suicide belief system and the cyclical nature of his suicidal behavior. Did he recognize that there were identifiable triggers, both internal (e.g., thoughts, images, feelings) and external, for his cyclical declines, many of which he could influence and target in therapy?

Cognitive therapy is about information processing, what we make of our experience. The patient's suicidal belief system is the articulation of his psychache. It is not just how and where he hurts, but how he has made sense of it. Can anything be done about it (helplessness)? Can it be tolerated (poor distress tolerance/psychache)? How are others affected (perceived burdensomeness)? Perhaps one of the more striking aspects of the interviews is the degree to which others take on his suicidal belief system, a significant liability in therapy if the belief system is not identified, targeted, and monitored. In each interview, the relative discusses the early onset of Arthur's problems and perceived deficiencies (unlovability), their chronic nature despite ongoing care (helplessness), the overwhelming nature of his pain (poor distress tolerance), and the growing burden in terms of time and energy (perceived burdensomeness).

Do I think the suicide could have been averted? Yes. Given that he was provided competent and appropriate care, what would I have done differently? I would have targeted his suicidal belief system more directly, coupled with traditional work, to enhance his distress tolerance. Oftentimes, a better understanding of the suicidal cycle enhances a sense of control and provides for related psychological needs (e.g., achievement, inviolacy, order, understanding), alleviating psychache enough to permit survival.

Suicide is about loss. Cognitive therapy for suicidality is about loss of perspective and understanding. The suicidal belief system provides a framework for understanding psychache and related psychological needs; it provides a way to restructure understanding and gain new perspectives. Even when the magnitude of pain seems overwhelming, there is opportunity for progress. As I read the interviews and the suicide note, I was struck by the potential for progress. But I muse that, as with every suicide, hindsight is twenty-twenty. I would like to have had the opportunity to have tried to save his life.

INTERVIEW WITH
THE PSYCHIATRIST

ESS: *The subject today is the tragic death of Arthur. As I understand it, you treated him for some time.*

MD: The circumstances were two suicides among present or recent medical students, which prompted the chairman to talk with me to see if we were missing something. In looking at it, medical students with problems were being treated by psychiatric residents, and we felt that they might not be able to pick up the subtleties that were required and, therefore, made a decision that all medical students and recent graduates would be treated by faculty. And so Arthur was the first patient that I saw under this program wherein only faculty members would treat young doctors. He was referred to me. He came in to see me, and I vividly remember his first visit because my impression was, clearly, that someday he was going to commit suicide.

ESS: *You had that as a gut feeling?*

MD: I was positive.

ESS: *Please tell me what clues you had.*

MD: Well, he comes in and tells me that the night before—he is very articulate—he was sitting in a chair, he wrapped cellophane around his face multiple times to suffocate himself, and the burning in his lungs got so bad that he ripped it off because the pain was so terrible; and that what he was planning for the night that I was seeing him was to repeat the cellophane, but he would duct tape his arms to the chair so that when the pain happened he wouldn't be able to extricate himself.

ESS: *Frightening.*

MD: Very frightening. And it was clear that—he gave a history—there were some psychosocial stressors, the breakup of a marriage, medical school, law school; but he was a very bright, articulate person who said to me, clearly, that, were he to get in the throes of depression again, he would kill himself because it was so unbearable. That first session I said to him, "I think there is hope." He had been managed medically—I think his ex-wife at the time gave him medications, and I said that, one, this is inappropriate, and, two, I'm going to do better medically than she has, and we'll find you the medicines, so I'll give you some hope from a medication standpoint. He was actively engaged in therapy with a therapist he had been seeing for a number of years by that time.

ESS: *His psychologist?*

MD: Yes. I increased his Effexor and then—I actually looked at his chart today—I called him a couple of times and got no answer. The question in my mind was: Did I need to hospitalize him? He was clear that I was welcome to hospitalize him, but if he were to get depressed again, if this didn't work, he was going to kill himself, whether that was after the hospitalization or not. So we didn't hospitalize him. I thought it was actually important to develop a working relationship with him in that period.

ESS: *How was he at that time?*

MD: He told me, and I quote, "I have every symptom in the book, except psychosis." And, really, my appointment with him at that time was to convince him and give him hope that there were still a lot of options regarding medication management, in addition to our continuing therapy, and he agreed. He had extreme concerns about confidentiality, and I reassured him that this does not go back to the school. I don't normally call patients after visits. I called him, it looks like, 18 days and then 19 days after, to check on how he was doing, because I had not heard from him, and obviously I was concerned. I didn't think he would kill himself then, but I knew he would kill himself. I knew it 100%. If you would have interviewed me then, I would have told you exactly that.

ESS: *Did you have a time frame?*

MD: Eventually, within 2 to 5 years; I didn't know the number, but he was clear. "I have depression. I can't go there again." And then, I was at that time using this system, it's pretty interesting now, especially with him, where, to get refills, he would call a telephone number and answer approximately 15 questions about his mood state and fifteen questions about his functioning state. The questions included: How many days in the last several days have you been depressed? How many days have you thought about suicide? I would get a score of how well he was doing from a depressive standpoint, how well he was doing from a life-functioning standpoint. That then gets faxed, and I would okay the refill, based on how he was doing. And he really did very well. The scores in the functioning are basically on a scale of o to 100, and his functioning scores were always in the 70s and 80s, at one point even 100, and his depression scores were very low, which is good; at one point even a 1, which is very good.

ESS: *Would that warrant a refill?*

MD: That means he got a refill every one of those months, and I'm counting about five months. And then one month, which is now three months after I saw him for the first time, he comes in, has no suicidal ideation, has no overt neurovegetative signs, an occasional return of symptoms—there had been a death, I think a grandfather had died. He continued therapy, and he talked about some side effects, sweating and premature ejaculation. So he has major depressive disorder, now with a good response. We again talked about what to do if the depression comes back, because this is what he is concerned about. We talked about medication. I stressed at that time the need for more careful follow-up, because it's been 3 months. He then goes 5 months and comes in at that time, because if you look here, for the first time his functioning score went from up in the 70s or 80s up to 100 down to 40, and his depression score went up to 18; so you see, he's getting worse. Well, when I saw he's getting worse, I check off the box, "No Refill"; [the] patient has to see me. He comes in.

ESS: *No automatic refill.*

MD: No automatic refill. Must make an appointment. And I have a note then, the last time I saw him; I saw him only three times. I asked the patient to come in because the telephone check score had decreased, and then he reports over the last few weeks that he's been bored with life, [finding it] hard to have pleasure, but had no return yet of suicidal ideation or suicide attempts; rather, there was kind of an emptiness that had developed in his life, and he had managed at that point to do his work. We continued the Effexor, and we added Wellbutrin to target some of the sexual side effects that he had. And then that is the last contact that I had with him in person, although later he returned back to absolutely ideal functioning, where his functioning scores go back up into the one hundreds and his depression goes back down to five and eight.

ESS: *Looking at that, you had no cause for alarm.*

MD: No cause for worry. I still would have told you that this guy is going to kill himself. I think I had been lucky that he responded well to some mild adjustments in medications. Then I got a phone message on my machine from another doctor that said something like: "Please give me a call. I have some bad news about a young doctor." Now, I've treated literally hundreds of medical people, but I knew that it was his death. I was positive. And he had really been completely fine under my watch, and then there was a certain perverse relief that his suicide did not happen under my watch because I think that would have been extremely difficult, more difficult for me than it was. Following this message, I called his mother and went to the house and visited with the family: mom, dad, sister, brother, and best friend. And the brother really looks like him and has the same voice. And I think that this meeting was as healing for the family, but it really helped me process it. The mom's question when I told her virtually exactly what I told you was, Why didn't anyone tell us that he was suffering this bad? The sad fact is, he was an adult, and we don't call moms and don't tell moms about their adult children.

ESS: *He was about 30.*

MD: Thirty-three. He was 28 when I saw him. We don't say your 28-year-old son is fine now, but he has a really bad mood disorder, and if it gets bad again, he might kill himself. I hope the meeting decreased some of their guilty feelings about having done enough or not having done enough. And then they also told me about some pretty significant attempts that I was not aware of, when he was younger, as a teenager or even as a child, when he had been pretty despondent. The thing that strikes me was that I knew and he knew, and I actually think we had a very strong relationship together in our brief time, because we didn't hide that. It was clear and we discussed it.

ESS: *Permit me to ask some further questions. What was his special quality that you talk about? What did he exude? What were those subtle signals? What was his pathology? Help me in this.*

MD: He was a mensch, so he was fun to be in the room with. He was a nice person. He was articulate.

ESS: *That doesn't presage suicide.*

MD: No. But I think that's important. He also was very articulate and was able to describe that he was clearly in his right mind, and in his right mind he was not going to suffer the depth of depression again, and that he had been there.

ESS: *But isn't the logic on the other side also, namely, he knew that he had come out of it?*

MD: No, but had you said that to him, it's clear that he would have said: "Of course I would come out of it again, but I don't want to be there again, and if I have to be there again, I would rather die." And he was clear on it.

ESS: *Is this a biological disorder in your opinion? Is it a psychodynamic process? Do we look to family dynamics? Is this a fellow who can't stand pleasure? He seems to have a peculiar, idiosyncratic, unique complex or disposition that he doesn't deserve happiness or success. He's phobic about being euphoric, about being pleasurable, a euphobia. He had it in adolescence. One of his worst days was when he returned from a summer camp. What happened there? He had a good time. And it opened the world to him that there were good times to be had, but they weren't for him. It wasn't that he had a bad time. A kind of perverse thing. Does any of this make sense?*

MD: It makes sense, but from my understanding of him, it doesn't describe him. He was petrified of his disorder and returning to it, and that it meant a model or scheme of his life invaded his thinking at all times. So there may have been where he would not want pleasure because it wouldn't last or he knew the pain was coming. But my sense was more than avoiding pleasure; he couldn't tolerate the pain of depression, and he knew it was coming.

ESS: *And what was this depression in his mind? Was it genetic, was it a biological curse?*

MD: It was a biological curse. Other psychosocial issues he was comfortable discussing, but that's not why he was spending time in the office with me, so our time was really focused. He wasn't avoiding those, but they were sort of compartmentalized—"that's being taken care of by the therapist"—but he did talk about relationships, about women, his difficulties there. But we really talked more about neurovegetative symptoms, suicidal ideation, and medication. So it's hard for me to give a psychodynamic explanation, because we didn't do psychodynamic work.

ESS: *What diagnosis would you give?*

MD: A depressive disorder without psychosis. He came in pretty depressed the first visit, and then he was fine for 2 years.

ESS: *Did you see that as cyclical?*

MD: He described it as cyclical—it's going to come back.

ESS: *A dicey question: What might have saved him?*

MD: Well, what might have saved him? I think, my sense is, that some of these cases are malignant, and there is nothing that will save them. I think my role is to provide all the options, and hope, and alternatives. But I don't think he was savable. I mean, how could I get a sense, after one visit, this guy is going to kill himself?

ESS: *Do you think that the physician should have been, might have been more proactive? Do you think you could have called him every fortnight? Do you think that might have helped, or would you have had to be very lucky and dropped in at the times when the depression was recurrent?*

MD: I don't think that would have helped. It wouldn't have helped during my watch, because he actually did really well during that period. And again, I'd say it was luck that he did well. It wasn't my skill, but with a little adjustment in medications and some hope, I think it was luck. Had he done his residency at my hospital, he would have killed himself, and I would have been his doctor. Either I would have done a telephone check—I mean it didn't matter, I could have called him every two weeks. He could have been in to see me for therapy and medications. He was going to kill himself when this came back.

ESS: *Could hospitalization have helped?*

MD: Again, no, there was no indication for hospitalization. It would have hurt. It would have hurt, during the time that I saw him. I don't know what would have happened. He was humiliated that he was even having to talk to a psychiatrist, that he was a student, that this was still going on. If he had been hospitalized, it would have been horrendous. I even talked to him about ECT.

ESS: *What did he say?*

MD: He was reasonable. He was talking like I was a colleague. He understood the disorder.

ESS: *Did he say, "If it's necessary, I'll undergo it?"*

MD: Absolutely. He didn't say, "No, I won't," he listened to it. I said, "Hey, you are ready to kill yourself, and you haven't tried half the things. We got all kinds of drugs, so we've got this med, that med, if that doesn't work, we could do ECT." We went over all the details of it.

ESS: *And he didn't say "Absolutely not?"*

MD: He was receptive. I wish that he had been offered ECT somewhere along the course. Again, he didn't need it during my little window with him, but if he went back and medications were pushed and that didn't work, ECT should have been part of the equation.

ESS: *Was he under treatment with anyone in the last months of his life?*

MD: I have no idea. I have no idea what happened to him after he graduated medical school and went on to law school. We, in psychiatry, don't talk about malignancy. Why can't we say not everyone with colon cancer lives? This guy had it bad, he died from it, and we do the best we can; and I'm telling you this was the clearest case of it I have ever seen of a psychiatric malignancy. He was persuaded that this was the way it was. "I have this thing and if it comes back, I'm going to kill myself. Actually I just did it last night, I tried it last night, I'm gonna try tonight." And the therapy was to say, "Hang on, give me a chance here and let me give you some hope." But he was right. You say no, I say yes. There is only so much one can do.

ESS: *You say he was bright, that he had conned himself.*

MD: There was no fight. I could fight all I wanted. He was clear. Even if he was illogical. This was fixed, this was immovable. He was stuck there. That's probably what said to me, "This guy is gonna do it." I could dance. It's not going to change his thinking, that "If I go back there, I can't tolerate it, I will kill myself." He didn't kill himself that night. So, I knew. I think I won. But the thing that I knew was he was going to win.

ESS: *Did you have a thought of referring him to someone?*

MD: I love referring patients out. We got the wise old men now. I'm happy to send that guy out to whoever those wise men are now. He didn't need them now, he was fine, he was asymptomatic, he was coming in to see me, he was seeing the therapist, he was fine. The question is, What was going to come? And it would have been a joke to send him to somebody. He would have said, "I have no symptoms. I got a little problem with ejaculation. My mood is good, my appetite. I'm fine." It wasn't a crisis, but I knew that it would come. He knew it would come. But I know he would have gotten worse, I would have picked it up, I would have done what I could, I would have sent him for a second opinion. We may have done hospitalization and ECT. We might have done perhaps much more aggressive treatment than maybe what happened where he went, I have no idea.

ESS: *And you would have saved his life for 5 years, let's say.*

MD: Yes, exactly. You know what, he would have moved somewhere else and killed himself. And I really felt, all we were doing was buying time. I think my role, and I believe this in my heart, is to fight as hard as I can against the patient's wish to be dead, and that's what I'm supposed to do.

CONSULTATION BY
AVERY WEISMAN, M.D.

Avery Weisman has been a miraculous person much of his life, and I view his beautiful essay, written at the age of 90, as a miracle in itself. Dr. Weisman is a rare creature: a serious student of philosophy. His first book was The Existential Core of Psychoanalysis *(1965). He has written several books, including two about the psychological autopsy:* The Psychological Autopsy *(1967), and* The Realization of Death: A Guide for the Psychological Autopsy *(1974). He spent most of his professional career in Boston, as professor of psychiatry at the Harvard Medical School; senior psychiatrist at the Massachusetts General Hospital; and principal investigator of Project Omega (a research study of how cancer patients cope with the illness and its ramifications) at the MGH. He is currently retired and lives in Scottsdale, Arizona. In my mind, he is the dean of American suicidology.*

What a waste of human potential!

This is an unusual psychological autopsy in that the significant others are so available, verbal, and articulate. The parents, siblings, best friend, ex-wife, and recent girlfriend added more information than is ordinarily reported in autopsy protocols.

According to those who should know, Arthur talked about his inevitable suicide from childhood on. This does not imply, however, that he was depressed from childhood on, although he was in psychotherapy for tantrums and so forth at an early age. Later, he was socially isolated, but then at some point he became very popular, with many friends. He married and divorced one woman and had an off-and-on affair with a girlfriend who became a source of information. In fact, overall, everyone had a positive view of Arthur, with minimal attention to how troublesome he must have been. During his short life, Arthur still managed to give ample promise of a productive life that he abnegated. His family was concerned and supportive, and this continued as long as Arthur allowed it.

Although Arthur was convinced about his grim fate and made numerous suicide attempts, the record of near misses is peculiar. As a pharmacist and physician, he had knowledge of toxicity and access to various drugs. Still, Arthur managed to postpone death until, of course, the final attempt, and even then he found the initial dose not enough to cause death.

Many years ago, I was a resident in pathology at the Boston City Hospital. I once asked Dr. Kenneth Mallory about the cause of death in a recent autopsy. He chided me gently and sagely: "We don't look for causes of death. We only find what a person died *with*, not *from*."

I certainly kept this in mind while trying to conduct psychological autopsies in the future. Because a psychological autopsy extends the range of a regular autopsy, it should also tell us what a person was like and lived *for*. This refers to values, aims, and the problems coped with. In order to flesh out the bare recital of disease or the surrounding facts of suicide, I therefore must make a distinction between *impersonal* information, shown by clinical, laboratory, and pathological findings; *interpersonal* information, which is usually called psychosocial; and the *intrapersonal* dimension, gained secondhand from survivors, that may reveal the dead person's inner life.

The immediate precipitants of suicide are almost as inaccessible as the private intrapersonal thoughts and feelings that push a reluctant person over the edge. Many illustrious people—a list too long to name individually—have committed suicide after overcoming extreme difficulties and calming down, only to take their lives during a period of relative quiescence. Whether they exchanged old problems for new ones is largely unknown, but they reportedly were calm and not manifestly depressed. Some people even feel very well before attempting suicide, a paradoxical event that is usually explained in a circular fashion as the decision to do it without further equivocation.

Why anyone kills himself or herself at a specific time is better not asked; it is tricky, enigmatic, and futile. In my clinical practice with patients of all sorts, the "why" question should never get an answer and should be understood not as a real question, but as an entreaty, appealing to a higher source for justification, such as, "Why me?" and "Why, oh why?"

Even for a hell-bent "malignant" suicide, timing is, in my opinion, a matter of conjecture and supposition. What remains is to piece together impersonal, interpersonal, and intrapersonal factors, likely to be fragmentary, but larded with our own prejudices and what we are pleased to call principles. Even wise old men, as we discussants are reputed to be, must be cautious in judgment. I like to believe that with collective experience, we can distinguish objective from subjective information, at least most of the time.

Psychological facts are, after all, not so much facts as low-level theories. Interviews with significant survivors after a death must be conducted circumspectly, allowing for idiosyncratic tendencies to idealize the dead, about whom nothing ill should be said. Not every report deserves equal credence. Some people will unwittingly cloak, rather than reveal, unpleasant and incriminating information. By selection, they have the most to lose and, therefore, are entitled to mitigate what they say. Nevertheless, it does not pay to be ultraskeptical, or we'd have nothing left. We can try to be discriminating and not take the survivors' agenda as factual all the time. As I read and reread these interviews by Dr. Shneidman, I found them honest but limited in how they wanted Arthur to be viewed in recollection. I noted very little grief, frustration, pity, or anger about the loss and suffering Arthur thrust upon them. The psychologist and the psychiatrist were very candid about deciding Arthur's risk but tended to treat him as a young colleague, not as a desperate patient.

At one time, I used to attend the so-called death conferences at the Massachusetts General Hospital. The medical staff met weekly to review deaths that had occurred since the last conference. The chief resident reviewed the history, medical course, tests, diagnosis, and final outcome before calling on other physicians and specialists who had been involved. I do not recall that nurses and social workers were ever asked for their reports, however lengthy their contact with the patient had been. Every death case was another instance of what this patient, a bearer of disease, died with. The ravages of the final and fatal disease were always depicted, with slides and laboratory data. Nothing besides the impersonal information was breached.

As a bystander, I wanted to interrupt and ask two questions: "Did you expect this patient to die when hospitalized?" and then, "What made you think so?" I never had the courage; the conference was speedy. I imagine that some doctors would have said, "Yes," and others, "No," and added a few words to address my second question. No one could be expected to say that they hadn't taken good care of the sick patient or that they might have done something else more effective. I think the conference would be aghast had the admitting doctor said that this patient had a malignant disease and was expected to die, anyway, regardless of what was done.

Suicide Evaluation

Assessing a suicide, before or after, involves two major considerations: risk factors and rescue factors. There are assorted factors on both sides, but not all those living alone in the central city or recently widowed should be found dead. Had he been admitted to a hospital for a medical illness, these statistical correlates alone would be unlikely to cause clinicians to set up suicide precautions. Nevertheless, numbers place him in a large group of potential suicides, even if he sits alone reading a newspaper in a dingy hotel lobby. However, a past history of suicide attempts, along with admission of depression, might be taken more seriously as a potential precipitant, especially if he talks about being better off dead. A clear plan pushes him further toward an imminent suicide risk, whereas indicators are calls to urgent rescue actions. Faltering in the drive to survive that ordinarily is hard to extinguish represents an immediate risk. The continuum of risk factors ranges from impersonal correlates to private intrapersonal dejection and suffering. Timing is only an approximation.

I am not aware of laboratory tests that unerringly identify acute suicide risk. The same is true for psychological inventories. In any event, shrewd clinical judgment is always needed. We note that euphemistic labels such as "chemical imbalance" are heeded more often than old-fashioned terms such as "bipolar disorder" or "depression without psychosis." I still wonder what triggers imbalance for people who seemingly get along and even thrive for years without an overt attempt. Must every suicide be preceded by depression? Or, given the relative success of antidepressants, do clinicians presume that there is some degree of depression behind every attempt? I yield to those with up-to-date skill in medicating depression and potential suicide. I beseech them to retain a regard for those of us born earlier who had little to offer besides a strong intention to preserve life.

Whereas risk factors are what potential suicides are endowed with, suffer from, and endure, rescue factors, or rescuability, are elements of a suicidal situation set up by the victim, who chooses the time, place, and significant others who might be alarmed enough to rescue him or her. Weisman and Worden (1972) described the Risk Rescue Rating, which assigns a numerical lethality for suicide attempts, not the lethality of intentions. However, with a good description of suicide planning, clinicians might also assess the rescue, as well as the risk, factors.

Rescue factors include treatment and management of lethality and the availability of supportive resources that can offer protection until the wave of intense suicidal lethality washes over. These factors have been reviewed so often that I may be excused from their reiteration. Treatment means such things as (1) psychotherapy of some kind, formal or impromptu, hortatory or permissive; (2) antidepressants; and (3) electroconvulsive therapy (ECT) for refractory cases (sometimes called malignant), along with a panoply of antipsychotic medications for those without other options.

Unless there lurks an undiscovered suicide chromosome in a depressive genetic cluster, medications seem to relieve depression but do not directly prevent suicide, except by spreading out the interval between attempts. I speak only from my grotto of retirement to ask if antidepressants distinguish between suicidal and nonsuicidal depression.

Supportive resources are supposed to be a good supplement for any treatment. Support is almost a cliché, as hardly anyone would advocate its opposite. If support fails, then we tend to call even dedicated efforts "interference" or "inappropriate intervention." Our clinical task is to define and describe support that is likely to succeed and to formulate plans for such vulnerable people as Arthur. Could anyone have targeted appropriate support for him? Of course, hospitalization, regardless of his objections, followed by consultation with a colleague familiar with ECT, constitute both treatment prospects and relevant support.

What About Arthur?

Arthur's risk factors and potential rescue factors scarcely need repetition. His risk factors are mainly lifelong preoccupation with suicide and his own demise, numerous attempts, intractable psychache, and unwavering certainty that life is frustration and death holds the only promise. Rescue factors include the significant others, Arthur's competence and undoubted success, and two skilled psychiatrists, one of whom was available for years and the other for the crucial period prior to death. As mentioned but not explained in the note, what were the periodic "boosts" that he dismissed as too temporary to matter? He claimed to feel so isolated, yet he is reported to have had many friends (how many does anyone need?) and close relations with at least two women, although he became scared of commitment when the relation became too much. This is hardly unusual. People evidently liked him; he was a "mensch," which is complimentary but hardly a preventative. He was fun to be with, it was said, despite gloominess inside.

One possible rescue factor was Arthur's unwillingness to take a lethal dose of whatever he ingested; he seems to have "failed" to die several times. This was an escape condition that he didn't take advantage of in his final attempt. He certainly knew the toxic amount, given his professional experience. Another rescue factor to consider was Arthur's abundant qualities that, just possibly, he could have used to reinforce the courage to cope and find meaning in his existence.

What else could therapists have done? Ron Maris said somewhere that most therapists secretly believe that they are able to save any suicidal patient. But when asked how they'd do it, they hesitate and stop short of a tangible remedy. At some frustrating point in psychotherapy, it is not uncommon to think about switching the patient to someone else. Here, too, there is silence about the qualifications of a new therapist—changing gender, age, training, and so forth all seem inadequate, even if we suppose that all our patients might be better off seeing someone else. Having a patient commit suicide must surely wound even the most cocksure therapist. Although I am sure that Arthur's psychiatrists were competent and conscientious, Arthur was asked about hospitalization and ECT, only to refuse. How urgently were these options recommended? Although he had attempted suicide by tape and asphyxiation just the night before, further avenues were discussed with him as if he were a rational colleague. Despite his being a mensch, I would have insisted on hospitalization and asked the help of an ECT colleague once Arthur was protected.

Arthur's suicide notes, although lengthy, seem very hollow at points. Wishing his survivors happiness in the future, in my opinion, was cruel. The idea of a celebration at some future time is particularly ironic.

I conclude with a word or two about the courage to cope with vulnerability in therapy. Quite apart from the antidepressants, which would help to a degree, learning how to cope effectively and to grapple with misfortune can be accomplished, even allowing for qualified skepticism. It is one thing to hope, but hope needs help and should be worked for. Despair needs help, too, with every means possible, when dealing with the enigma of suicide.

LETTER TO THE MOTHER

[Date]

Mrs. Hannah Zukin

Dear Mrs. Zukin:

Here we are, practically at the end of this journey, in which I have tried to generate substantial information about the death of your son with the hope that you will find some new helpful insights and some anchors of solace. If one produces enough rich ore, there ought to be some valuable nuggets within it. You must know that I have had high regard and affection for you right from the beginning, and I hope you won't find it inappropriate if I say that this is my special letter to you.

Please let me go directly to what is at the forefront of my thoughts.

Language does not permit me to express the depth of my sorrow for your loss. As you know, I am a father and a grandfather. As a whole, my life has been blessed by luck, but it is fair to say that we have had our vicissitudes, some of them quite serious and threatening. I don't know what I would have done or how I could have survived if one of my loved ones had committed suicide. It is, alas, easy for me to cry for your anguish. From the beginning, this project has been a labor admixed with pain.

In all candor, I don't see what I could have done that I don't ordinarily (or even extraordinarily) do. I don't see what I might have done that your son wouldn't have trumped. His pain and narcissism were more potent than my benign expertise, even at its most active. Looking you in the eye, I cannot honestly say that *I* would have saved him, but I can swear to you that I would have tried my best to keep him alive. And perhaps I would have been more draconian than those who treated him. But that is hindsight, and hindsight is not only clearer than perception-in-the-moment but also unfair to those who actually lived through the moment. In the end, Arthur marshaled and focused all his considerable strengths to his deathful purpose. His assets were the tools of his undoing. Suicide is winning the hand but being unable to walk away from the table—and plunging the entire room into unexpected and pervasive sorrow.

After 50 years of suicidological practice, I have to confess to myself that there are some few people who have a combination of intense psychological pain and a low threshold for absorbing it—and who seem doomed from an early age. I am not sure that even Frieda Fromm-Reichman or Marguerite Sechahaye—legendary therapists of difficult patients—working together could have saved Arthur. But I want to reserve the delusion that he would not die under my care. I believe I could save from suicide any person with whom I choose to work and who chooses to work with me, including in that choice that person's strong positive transference to me as a life-saving figure. I must take this position if I am to bring anyone ashore.

I call my mode of therapy *anodyne therapy*. Of course, I recognize that the key purpose of any psychotherapy is anodynic—to reduce the patient's pain. But what I think is crucial here is the conscious focus of the therapist on the psychic pain (psychache), on the reduction and mollification of that pain, combined with the necessary redefinition and reconceptualization of that pain as somehow bearable after all. And further, anodyne therapy places a fresh template in the therapist's mind that focuses on the patient's frustrated psychological needs as the malignant foundation or source of the patient's psychache. If the individual needs to stop certain pains in order to continue to live, then it follows that those pains need to be addressed, reduced, and redefined so that the urge to self-destruction can be put aside. I am unapologetic about the Melvilleian tone of this paragraph, for I believe that many of the roots of suicide and many of the clues to prevention are to be found in the intellectual bomb bursts of the Melville canon. For what is suicide but a damp and dismal November in the mind?

Speaking of Melville, Arthur suffered from what I'll call a *Redburn complex*. *Redburn* is Melville's third novel, written in 1849, when Melville was still in his 20s, about a young man who, from early childhood, is embittered and taught, so he thinks, by life's lessons to be pessimistic and dour. He tends to be self-abnegating; he sees the cup of life as more than half suffering rather than more than half pleasure. These negative life orientations come in early and stick to the ribs. Melville knows the rigor of life's winter months. Here is Redburn:

> Cold, bitter cold as December, and bleak as its blasts, seemed the world then to me; there is no misanthrope like a boy disappointed; and such was I, with the warm soul of me flogged out by adversity. . . . Talk not of the bitterness of middle age and after life; a boy can feel all that and much more, when upon his young soul the mildew has fallen; and the fruit, which with others is only blasted after ripeness, with him is nipped in the first blossom and bud. And never again can such blights be made good; they strike in too deep, and leave such a scar that the air of Paradise might not erase it.

So Arthur, from boyhood on, is a secret Redburn, suffering wherever he went. Therapists from heaven—Paradise itself—might not have been able to save him.

As a psychotherapist I have an ingrained responsibility to be empathic, to resonate to Arthur's private psychological pain, and to reaffirm his right to end his suffering. But at the same time, in this same role, I am aware of his towering narcissism, his view that his suffering is somehow unique, that he is special among men—a kind of malignant grandiosity that asserts that no one has ever had it as bad as he has. This almost delusional greatness-of-*my*-pain seems to be present in many suicidal people.

In the grisly postmortem spin-the-bottle game played among survivors—to see to whom the neck of the bottle points as having been conspicuously derelict or guilty or culpable or negligent or unfeeling in relation to the suicide victim—we tend to forget that the decedent is also a player. Each person who commits suicide must, willy nilly, take some responsibility for his own death. Suicide is a self-inflicted death. We are entitled to be critical of Arthur for his self-centered and shortsighted act. *De mortuis nihil nisi bonum* ("Of the dead [speak] nothing but good.") In a psychological autopsy, the gloves are off, and we must speak candidly about the deceased. If our accounts were limited to "nothing-but-good," then we would be giving a eulogy and not conducting an autopsy. I might have helped Arthur while he was alive—I would have broken my back trying—but I need to say I don't like him dead. Years ago I wrote that the suicidal person puts his psychological skeleton in his survivor's closet. It's not a pretty picture. Perhaps that is why the early Freudians (around 1910) saw suicide primarily as hostility toward the parents: It appeared to them that in assuaging his own desperate need to stop the unbearable psychological pain, the suicidal person, coincidentally at least, broke his mother's heart. We see that Arthur, for all his wit, cannot escape inflicting collateral damage on his family. Part of our discomfort in this case has to do with our puzzlement over how he could be so thoughtless. The answer, I believe, lies in the constriction, the concentration, the tunneling of vision, the pathological narrowing and focus on the Self that is a usual part of the suicidal state. Boris Pasternak, the famous author, writing of the suicide of several young Russian poets, put it this way:

> A man who decides to commit suicide puts a full stop to his being, he turns his back on his past, he declares himself bankrupt and his memories to be unreal. They can no longer help or save him, he has put himself beyond their reach. The continuity of his inner life is broken, and his personality is at an end. And perhaps what finally makes him kill himself is not the firmness of his resolve but the unbearable quality of this anguish which is empty because life is stopped and he can no longer feel it. (Pasternak, 1959)

Seeing him this way, I might have, in psychotherapy with him, focused on his frustrated psychological need for inviolacy. The need for inviolacy relates to the need to protect the self, to maintain one's psychological space, to remain separate, independent, unfettered, left alone to be loved but not necessarily required to love back—a "knock before entering" sign on the door to one's psyche. Inimically, he kept people out, and yet he desperately needed them. Inviolacy is obviously related to the psychological needs for autonomy, achievement, and counteraction. I asked Arthur's former wife, a physician herself, to rate Arthur's investments among 20 possible psychological needs, using 100 points. She deposited all 100 chips on just one of his needs: inviolacy. One could predict that Arthur might go from medical specialty to medical specialty, even from profession to profession (let's try law); from one significant other to another; from one set of criticisms to another; always driven by a need to find a safe Self that he could never quite formulate. He and I might have read H. L. Mencken together. I would know that we were making progress when Arthur called me one of Mencken's favorite terms, a "boob." And when Mencken failed to hold our interest sufficiently, we might move on to Melville. Melville is profound and dour enough to keep anyone alive for years—except his own eldest son. I would not have tried to change Arthur's character; just extend its duration. We would learn together that not even he was more complicated and more layered and inwardly benighted than Captain Ahab and that there is more than one way of staying afloat in the vast Pacific of life.

Simultaneously, we would come to know that the quantity of Arthur's pain was not unique, that others have hurt as much and suffered as grievously and have continued to endure. Together, he and I would redefine and fine-tune our understanding that, in actual practice, "unbearable" and "intolerable" really mean barely bearable and somehow tolerable, and that these terms can be incorporated into a dour pattern for life-long survival. Hopefully, he could come to do what Emperor Hirohito ordered his overwhelmed people to do at the end of World War II: to suffer the unsufferable and to endure the unendurable—and to live.

Concomitantly, our therapy would continuously focus on the sources of his psychache, namely the frustration of his contradictory psychological needs for inviolacy, achievement, order and succorance. And, of course, I would have sought out consultation and support from my experienced friends some of whom you have already met in this volume. Saving a human life is a complicated mission.

So in the end we see that there is no simple understanding of any one suicide, that we are back at the end of *Rashomon*, scratching our heads, wanting to run the film over again albeit with a different ending, and, unhappily, thinking about it and puzzling over it for the rest of our lives as to who and what played this or that role in the tragic ending and whether Arthur was star-crossed from early on. Genes and fortune bent Arthur to this end, chronically skating near the precipices of the deep canyons of life, and one day tripping and falling in.

With every best personal wish for your health, your welfare, and your indomitable spirit.

Sincerely,

Edwin S. Shneidman, Ph.D.
Professor of Thanatology Emeritus, UCLA

APPENDIX
ARTHUR'S SUICIDE NOTE

All I do is suffer each & every day. Every moment is pain or numbness. How long can one go without pleasure. I guess these will really be my last words. I've written like this literally dozens of times before.

I would like to address every person I know individually, but as a person who doesn't care about anything, I guess it's difficult to care enough to spend the time to do that.

Thank you everyone who has tried to help me over the years. You know who you are. Don't feel you failed. I guess this was inevitable. The suffering needs to be relieved.

Depression has slowly eaten away at my life while I've continued to somehow function, make it through school & work, it has only been by an inch that I've hung in there to not fall out or get fired.

I've jeopardized my career more times than anyone could imagine. I've tossed friends and friendships to the side as the years have passed, and this has taken a great toll on me without anything giving me pleasure in life. I found few people who either occasionally gave me some joy, or I was originally comfortable with them relative to my discomfort with the rest of the world.

I have avoided mentioning anyone by name because again I cannot bear to address all. My thoughts continually come to 2 individuals though, [Pal] and [girlfriend].

[Pal], I love you and am sorry for leaving you in this way. I am sorry for leaving you. You are strong. You will survive without me. Thank you for everything.

[Girl], thanks for the comfort and pleasures we had when we were together. Thanks for your patience and caring for me. I am sorry, so sorry for all the times I hurt you. Be happy. I wish you a life of happiness.

I am going to get to go to sleep, to feel calmness and peace. I won't have to struggle with another day.

[Sis], I am so sorry for leaving you with the burden of the loan you took out for me. I wish I could change this. Please understand I had every intention of taking care of the loan. Please take my car or whatever else and use that if you can. Thank you also for all of your support over the years. You are/have been a great little sister. Hang in there. Understand that I was just suffering too much to bear anymore. I love you.

[LATER]

It's over. Finally over. I will do it now. I have nothing left. My mind is racked with thoughts. I can't concentrate or perform at work. Work is far too demanding a field for someone in my current condition. I could keep going through the motions. Anyway, it is not this that is ending it for me. It is the last years that I have managed to slowly ruin my life. I couldn't hold it together long enough anymore to put myself in position to give me the small boosts that used to get me over this type of despair.

I have thought about suicide and contemplated doing it thousands of times in my life. No one should feel they failed. I could not be saved I guess.

[11:30 P.M.]

I am getting very drowsy. I will likely fall asleep soon. I hope I have taken enough to finish this. I would not want to be revived or survive through this. It would only make life more horrific to deal with. Please do not resuscitate me if alive when found. *Please.*

NO AUTOPSY. Leave my body alone.

I did it with primarily crushed Oxycontin placed into capsules. I crushed it some time ago so can't remember how many mg's but I think it should do the trick. . . .[1]

---

[1]*Arthur's medications:* Two years before Arthur's death, he saw a physician who—having diagnosed him with major depressive disorder, recurrent, severe—prescribed Effexor, 100 mg. Subsequently, his wife (also a physician) prescribed Prozac, 10–40 mg, but it was not effective. She then prescribed Wellbutrin, 300 mg, which was also ineffective. A year later, when he was hospitalized, he was again prescribed Effexor, 75–150 mg, and, in addition, Eskalith (lithium carbonate), 450 mg, and Celexa, 40 mg.

I'm alert, but I just feel like shit. I want to get this over with. I just want to take meds so I will go unconscious before I go but it is getting difficult to do in this condition.

Vomited. Damn it. I just threw up a shitload of lithium.

There were many other family members and friends that I deeply love and have cherished but again many that I will not individually address. You have been in my heart and thoughts frequently over the years and now even if I have been bad at keeping in touch.

Please DONATE MY ORGANS if possible.

If I were to drop out now wait til hear from university. If get in then I am set. I can fuck up as much as I want without grave consequences. Don't need to impress anyone. Just seem to get my license and keep passing through. . . .

It has been over 13 years since my first attempt at suicide. Although I was the one who ultimately aborted, I can earnestly say that it was not crying out for help. I had every intention of only avoiding further pain which I knew I was inevitably going to experience.

At that time I withstood immense torture day after day in high school. No one was cruel to me but I lived in isolation. I did not adjust to the school, and therefore sat alone in the hallways or in the library during break times.

I thought of suicide frequently, but the decisive instigator was an extremely unexpected & unlikely one. What occurred was a weekend of *normalcy*. I went to a camp weekend & found myself socializing with a popular group of kids & even catching the eye of a girl. On coming home, I could not imagine handling the contrast that was in store for me when I returned to school the next day.

At that time I had already heard the phrase "Suicide is a permanent solution to a temporary problem." I believed this and believed that surely one day in the not too distant future I would have a social life I enjoyed, a spouse, family & career. I did not want to go through the tortuous days, weeks, months, or even years that were going to occur before this though.

Somehow I made it through that period. I even ended up achieving most of what I knew would be coming my way one day. By the end of high school I had a large group of friends, a list of girlfriends, and to others a bright future ahead of me.

Well, that did not last. My periods of success in life have definitely been there, however my periods of despair have sadly been there in much greater strength and preponderance.

I ultimately skipped on the permanent solution to my supposedly temporary problem. But I am here today and for too many days in the past, I am seeing that my problems were not as "temporary" as I imagined. On the other hand, they are quite permanent. They are within me. I cannot hide from them, or shake them with any success.

I have gone through literally countless years of therapy & now over 2 years of antidepressant medications. Why is it that I should believe that one day I will be "happy." It now more than ever appears that I will spend my life jumping from short periods of pleasure to tremendously long periods of pain. When I now look into the future I do not see myself at one time achieving happiness in my life. When I think of myself as a 50, 60, 70, or even 80 year old man I imagine that I will experience huge periods of depression, just as I have been having at this moment. Regardless of what anyone else claims, that would not be a life which had been worth living.

I do not wish that I could hang around for a while. I feel that I am a decent person, and actually have much to offer others. I believe that I could be a terrific and compassionate physician and have an extremely successful career. That is all only possible though if I can be content in my life outside of work (which I don't see possible).

I want so badly to be back with [my girlfriend]. We had something so special. We understood each other and cared immensely for each other. I just miss her so much right now. Thinking of her & my loss of her gives me a heavy feeling in my chest as I write this. Why did I ever break up with her then? Well, I again was not content with my life. I guess I have always dreamt of myself as a savior being someone who would physically drag her off and force me into environments which were good for me & lead me to pleasures in my life. My pathology was too strong for this though. I was not happy and felt there may be a woman out there that could just render me completely content with all of my life.

So now I'm hungry out here alone. I cannot leave my apt. I cannot see myself finding a more terrific woman than she is. However, I feel that going back to her just may not be an option at this time. I also fear, and believe, that if we were to go back together we would go through another honeymoon period, and then I would end up unhappy again several months later.

I do not want to torture her. I care about her & want the rest of her life to be a happy one. Right now I am so torn. I am sinking. I am in the ocean drowning. She is all I feel can save me. The chances of me bringing her down with me are too strong though.

If I go this evening, then I go to spare her more unnecessary pain, & to avoid our inevitable cycle of torture. I will be unhappy ultimately regardless of whether I drag her down with me.

My baby. I can't write to you. I just want to express myself to you by holding you, scratching your back & rubbing your legs. I want to smile at you, and see your beautiful smile back to me. You are strong. I know you are a survivor, and will come through this. I do worry tremendously for you though. In many ways I would like to say untruths to you so that it would be easier for you to move on, I cannot though. The thought of our openness and honesty is a single pleasure which I need so much to have with me as I leave this world. You go ahead and take your wonderful qualities to someone else though. It would not be a betrayal of my & my memory. I want your happiness. If there is anything above when we are gone, then I will be smiling at you as a close friend when I see you happy in your life. Marry and raise a family. I will feel happy to be watching your children as any uncle would.

Bye baby.

To [my pal]: You have been my best friend ever. You have been my confidant, support, and joy for a long time now. I cannot express how much our friendship has meant to me. I thank you for all of the good times we've had, and for all of the support you have given me. You are a terrific person, and will do great in life. I know that my departure will be a terrible blow, but please move on and make a marvelous life for yourself. You can keep me in [your] heart & know that you were always there for me and appreciated. Have a drink on my birthday, remember me and be happy for me. Please be happy for me because I no longer must feel the pain that I have for so long had.

These comments go for all of those who would claim to love or care for me. Please don't consider my departure a tragic life lost which could have been wonderful. Please, I beg you to celebrate for me that I can be free of pain.

[Brother]: Keep on trucking. You've obviously done a great job this year. I know that we suffer from some similar pathology, but I believe that you will be able to find that right woman to share your life with. I wish that we could have grown old together around the Scrabble board.

ARTHUR'S SUICIDE NOTE

I would write to others such as my mother, father, grandparents, aunt, cousin, but I must get on with my plans before it becomes too late in the night. Too many times I have been close to this point and just fell asleep, each time awakening to face another day of pain. Finally I would like to avoid that additional day of pain.

My illness is a tragedy, but it is one that I unfortunately cannot overcome. Those that tried to help me, including my therapist, should not feel that they failed. He and many others made my life more bearable in many ways. I have learned much about myself in the last 2–3 years and am finally at a place where I actually know myself, like myself, and am perhaps as close to my highest level of functioning as possible.

Life is not all that people crack it up to be. I have always said "Ignorance is bliss. I wish I was ignorant." Oh do I wish I was in a simple world where my only needs were food, shelter & clothing, and not some deep spiritual satisfaction.

I will die tonight, or I will call my sweetheart and most likely die another night, but also have dragged her through more nightmare.

[Sis]: I am sorry for the pain I have caused you so many times in your life, & now again. You are a wonderful person with immense potential. You will be the best social worker and bring incredible things to all who touch you. As I said earlier, please understand that this is what I needed for me. I need you to be happy that I'm out of pain. I feel terrible about the debt that I will be leaving you with. My student loans. I apologize. Please take all of my property, my car, and the money in my checking account. (Dad, I beg of you to help her with this debt. Please do not allow my death to put a financial burden on her which could hold her back for years to come.)

REFERENCES

American Psychiatric Association. (1994). *Diagnostic and Statistical Manual of Mental Disorders. Fourth Edition.* Washington, D.C.: American Psychiatric Association.

Attwater, D. (1965). *The Penguin dictionary of saints.* Baltimore: Penguin Books.

Bridges, P. K., Bartlett, J. R., Hale, A. S., Poynton, A. M., Malizia, A. L., & Hodgkiss, A. D. (1994). Psychosurgery: Stereotactic subcaudate tractomy. An indispensable treatment. *British Journal of Psychiatry, 16,* 599–611; discussion 612–613.

Brown, G., Linnoila, M., and Goodwin, F. (1992). Impulsivity, aggression, and associated affects: Relationship of self-destructive behavior and suicide. In Maris. R., Berman, A. L., Maltsberger, J. T. and Yufit, R. (Eds.), *Assessment and Prediction of Suicide.* New York: Guilford Press.

Curphey, T. J. (1961). The role of the social scientist in the medicolegal certification of death from suicide. In N. L. Farberow & E. S. Shneidman (Eds.), *The cry for help.* New York: McGraw-Hill.

Hollis, C. (2003). Developmental precursors of child- and adolescent-onset schizophrenia and affective psychoses: Diagnostic specificity and continuity with symptom dimensions. *British Journal of Psychiatry, 182,* 37–44.

Kanner, L. (1943). Autistic Disturbances of Affective Contact. *The Nervous Child, 2,* 217–250.

Kramer, P. (1993). *Listening to prozac.* New York: Viking.

Litman, R. E., Curphey, T. J., Shneidman, E. S., Farberow, N. L., & Tabachnick, N. (1963). Investigations of equivocal suicides. *Journal of the American Medical Association, 184,* 924–929.

Maris, R. (1981). *Pathways to suicide.* Baltimore: Johns Hopkins University Press.

Maris, R., Berman, A. L., and Silverman, M. (2000). *Comprehensive textbook of suicidology*. New York: Guilford Press.

Murray, H. A. (1938). *Explorations in personality*. New York: Oxford University Press.

Neugebauer, R., & Reuss, M. L. (1998). Association of maternal, antenatal and perinatal complications with suicide in adolescence and young adulthood. *Acta Psychiatrica Scandinavica, 97,* 412–318.

Pasternak, B. (1959). *I remember: Sketches for an autobiography*. New York: Pantheon.

Rudd, M. D., Joiner, T. E., & Rajab, M. H. (2000). *Treating suicidal behavior: An effective time-limited approach*. New York: Guilford Press.

Shneidman, E. (1971). Suicide among the gifted. *Suicide and Life-Threatening Behavior,* 1 (1), 23–45. Reprinted in A. Leenaars (Ed.), *Lives and deaths: selections from the works of Edwin S. Shneidman*. Philadelphia: Brunner/Mazel.

Shneidman, E. (1973). Suicide notes reconsidered. *Psychiatry, 36,* 379–395.

Shneidman, E. S. (1977). The psychological autopsy. In L. I. Gottschalk, et al. (Eds.), *Guide to the investigation and reporting of drug abuse deaths* (pp. 179–210). Washington, DC: Government Printing Office; reprinted in A. A. Leenaars (Ed.). (1999). *Lives and deaths: Selections from the works of E. S. Shneidman*. Philadelphia: Brunner/Mazel.

Shneidman, E. (1979). A bibliography of suicide notes, 1856–1979. *Suicide and Life-Threatening Behavior, 9,* 57–59.

Shneidman, E. (1980). *Voices of death*. New York: Harper & Row.

Shneidman, E. (1993) *Suicide as psychache*. Northvale, NJ: Aronson.

Shneidman, E. (1993). An example of a death clarified in a court of law. *In Suicide as Psychache*. Northvale, NJ: Aronson. Reprinted in A. Leenaars (Ed.), *Lives and deaths*. Philadelphia: Brunner/Mazel.

Shneidman, E., & Farberow, N. (1957a). Some comparisons between genuine and simulated suicide notes. *Journal of General Psychology, 56,* 251–256.

Shneidman, E., & Farberow, N. (Eds.). (1957b). *Clues to suicide*. New York: McGraw-Hill.

Stacey, P. (2003). Floor time. *The Atlantic Monthly*, Jan/Feb, 127–134.

Stoff, D. M., & Mann, J. J. (1997). The neurobiology of suicide. *Annals of the New York Academy of Sciences* (Vol. 836). New York: New York Academy of Sciences.

Weisman, A. D. (1974). *The realization of death: A guide for the psychological autopsy*. New York: Behavioral Publications.

Weisman, A., and Worden, W. (1972). Risk-rescue rating in suicide assessment. Archives of *General Psychiatry, 26,* 553–560.

Zetzel, E. (1965). Depression and the incapacity to bear it. In M. Schur (Ed.), *Drives, behavior* (Vol. 2, pp. 243–274). Madison, CT: International Universities Press.

Zhang, J., et al. (2002). Studying suicide with psychological autopsy. *Suicide and Life-Threatening Behavior, 32* (4), 370–379.

INDEX

Fromm-Reichman, Frieda, 160

Genetics, 27, 39, 87, 94, 133–138, 163
Girlfriend, interview with, 115–124
Goodwin, F., 101
Grandiosity, 47, 88, 89, 90, 101, 159, 161

Hemingway, E., 101
Hirohito (Emperor of Japan), 163
Hodgkiss, A.D., 89
Hollis, C., 87
Hopelessness, 138
Hospitalization, 16, 19, 20, 144, 150, 156
Huxley, A., 103

Inviolacy, need for, 140, 162

Jael, 85
Jamison, Kay, 103
Joiner, T.E., 138
Jung, C.G., 99

Kanner, L., 53n
Kramer, P., 100
Kurosawa, A., 32

Learning disability, 15, 24, 50, 51, 60, 87
Letter to mother, 159–164
Linnoila, M., 101
Litman, R.E., 33, 45–48
Lobotomy, 9
Loneliness, 20, 41
Loss, 106, 141

Mallory, K., 152
Maltsberger, J.T., 85–90
Mann, J.J., 87
Maris, R., 99–103, 156

Medications, 16, 28, 43, 47, 51, 52, 55, 56, 65, 66, 79, 80, 93, 100, 103, 131, 133, 144, 145, 146, 155, 166n
Melville, H., 160, 161, 163
Mencken, H.L., 163
Menninger, K., 100
Method of Difference, 4, 7
Mifune, T., 32
Mill, J.S., 4, 7
Mother, interview with, 23–29
Motto, J., 49–57
Murray, H.A., 138

Narcissism. See grandiosity
Needs, psychological, 160
Neugebauer, R., 87

Orestes, 86

Pain and psychache, 8, 20, 36, 41, 42, 47, 49, 54, 61, 75, 77, 81, 86, 90, 100, 110, 113, 121, 135, 137, 138, 147, 156, 159, 160
Pal, interview with, 91–98
Pasternak, B., 162
Pelagia (Saint), 3n
Perfectionism, 17, 81, 88, 101
Pessimism, 4, 95, 97, 110, 131
Physician, interview with, 143–150
Plath, Sylvia, 100
Psychache. See pain
Psychological autopsy, 11, 12, 31, 33, 46, 152, 161
Psychotherapist, interview with, 125–136
Psychotherapy, 50, 51, 54, 66, 79, 80, 81, 122, 125

Rage. See anger
Rajab, M.H., 138
Rankin, J., 4

ABOUT THE AUTHOR

Edwin Shneidman, Ph.D., was born in 1918 in York, Pennsylvania. He is professor emeritus of thanatology at the University of California, Los Angeles. He served in World War II, advancing from private to captain. In the 1950s he was cofounder and codirector of the Los Angeles Suicide Prevention Center, with Norman Farberow and Robert Litman. In the 1960s he was the chief of the Center for Study of Suicide Prevention at the National Institute of Mental Health in Bethesda, Maryland. He has been visiting professor at Harvard University and at the Ben Gurion University of the Negev in Beersheva. He has been a research associate at the Karolinska Hospital in Stockholm and a fellow at the Center for Advanced Study in the Behavioral Sciences at Stanford University. In 1968, he founded the American Association of Suicidology. He is the founding editor of the quarterly journal *Suicide and Life-Threatening Behavior*. He has been editor or coeditor of a dozen books. He is the author of *Deaths of Man* (nominated for a National Book Award), *Voices of Death*, *Definition of Suicide*, *The Suicidal Mind,* and *Comprehending Suicide* (winner of a CHOICE Award). He is widowed and has four sons (all health professionals) and six grandchildren.

CPSIA information can be obtained at www.ICGtesting.com
Printed in the USA
BVOW082313080412

286784BV00011B/3/P

9 780195 172737